Goldie!

A day in the life of a blind dog

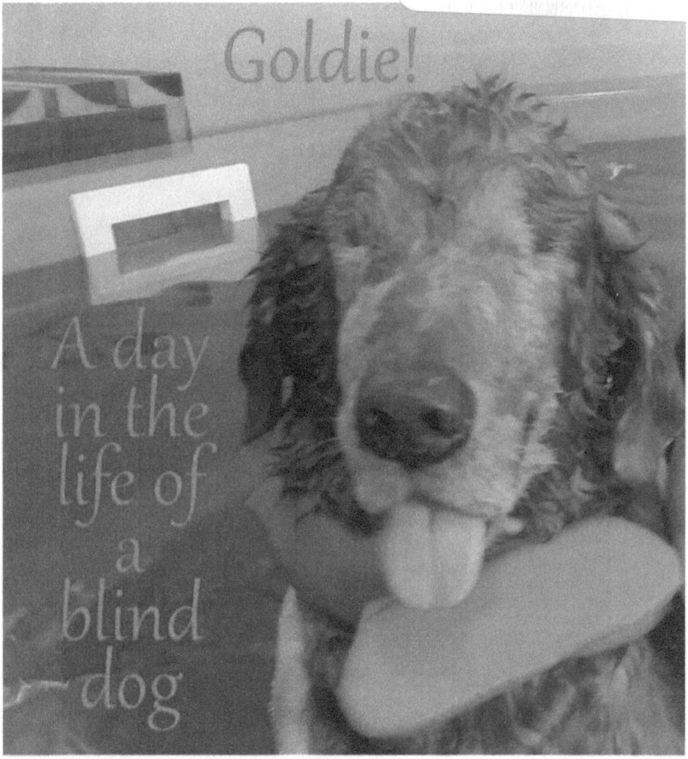

Copyrighted Material

Copyrighted © 2018 Elizabeth Parker

All rights reserved. No part of this publication may be reproduced or transmitted in any form by any means, electronic or mechanical, including photocopy, recording, or any information storage and retrieval system, without permission in writing from the publisher.

Real names may have been changed or omitted to protect the individual's privacy.

Please note that this book is not meant to be utilized as a training manual, nor is it meant to advise on how to train any dog. Please follow the instructions of a professional dog trainer if you are seeking assistance with your dog. Thank you.

First Edition

ISBN: 9781790830626

Hardcover ISBN: 9798757260310

A portion of the proceeds from the sales of this book will be donated to an animal rescue group.

Just a heartfelt thank you to all of the doctors and veterinary technicians who put their heart into their work and their patients.

My love to Goldie who has taught me so much about life in just a few short years. Life isn't always easy; however, perseverance goes a very long way.

Thanks to both Duke and Ginger for being so very patient with Goldie even as she stumbled on top of them often! Duke, my heart, I miss you boy!!

Along those same lines, thank you to my mother who was instrumental in helping me with Goldie on the day I brought her home from the hospital and the days that followed. And I'm sure Goldie thanks you too for all of her "get well" toys!

Thank you to my niece who rose up to the challenge of trekking across the country with Goldie and me! We had many long conversations and so many laughs. I love you!

Table of Contents

Goldie's Note: 6

The Human Author's Note: 10

Chapter 1-Glaucoma 14

Chapter 2-The Search Begins 20

Chapter 3-GOLDIE! 28

Chapter 4-Facing the Truth 36

Chapter 5-Home Sweet Homecoming 60

Chapter 6- Coping with Blindness 76

Chapter 7-Just a Normal Day 84

Chapter 8-Duke 88

Chapter 9 -Vegas! 98

Chapter 10-Don't Move That! 110

Chapter 11 -Introducing People 118

Chapter 12-Ginger! 126

Chapter 13-Blind dogs CAN swim! 134

Chapter 14-A Thread of Awareness 144

Extras to remember 152

Dog Sitters 158

Goldie's Note:

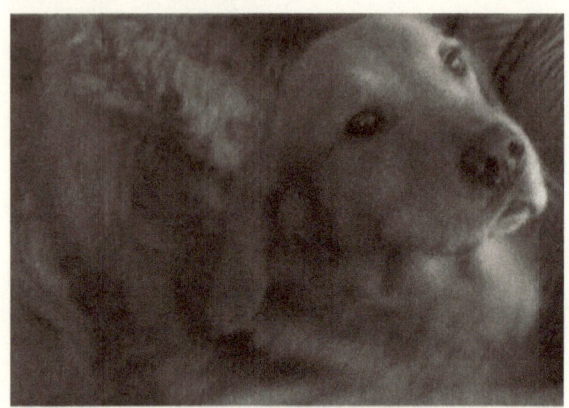

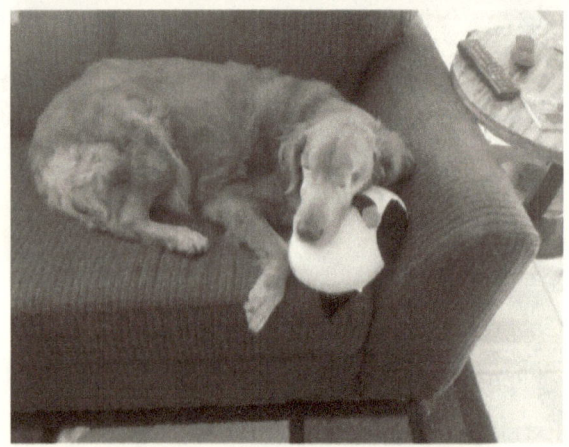

Mom always grabs the computer and says she's busy penning her next novel. She tries her best to ignore me as I slap her on the wrist with my paw, or get up and grab a toy. She thinks I just want attention. But honestly, all I wanted to do is tell MY story. So, this time, I decided to be persistent and chose not to be ignored. Finally, I get to write a book of my own.

Ok, well maybe my mom is writing it on my behalf.

See, not only do I not have thumbs, which makes it difficult to type, but I'm also blind. Oh, and I'm also a dog. Or so I've been told.

I, on the other hand, think of myself as a bit human. But that's another story.

I wanted to share my story with other pups just like me because the journey I've been on wasn't an easy one. She tells me I'm one of the ambassadors for blind dogs, but I'm sure there are other dogs just like me with their own unique victories. High paw to all of you out there!

But as mom says, I'm a trooper. Oh, and Mom also calls me Goldie girl, Goldielocks, Goldalishish, a champion, cutest girl in the world, and sometimes she even has the audacity to call me a bad girl, but I yell at her for that. You can catch a video of that on mom's social media, I'm sure.

I hope this book helps you and your pup. Tell them I'm rooting for them!

Okay, Mom is grabbing the computer from me. Gotta go. Here's my story!

Love, Goldie

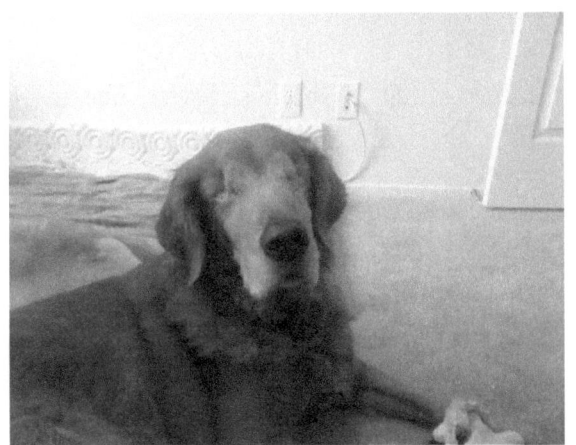

The Human Author's Note:

I wanted to share Goldie's journey because I believe there are other people like me, who have a dog they love with all of their heart. A dog who is blind or going blind. Goldie battled with glaucoma, but other illnesses cause blindness as well. Regardless of the cause, the result is the same; blindness.

It's a frightening experience if you've never dealt with it before. There are instances, situations and little tweaks here and there that need to be made. Something that you may never realize when your dogs have their eyesight. I never realized any of these things until I had a blind dog.

When I was deciding whether to have Goldie's eyes enucleated, I've heard some helpful and encouraging comments. However, I had also listened to others who advised that it might be better to have Goldie euthanized. Their reasoning? A blind dog will suffer and not enjoy life.

I'm here to tell you that nothing is farther from the truth.

I am thankful that I had enough wits about me, and enough logic, (along with long conversations with doctors) to ignore the comments about having Goldie euthanized.

That would have been one decision I would have regretted for the rest of my life.

Is life with a blind dog different? Sure, a little. But honestly, most of the time I forget she is blind.

As a matter of fact, so do others who meet her. They often do a double take and zoom in closer with their own eyes to notice Goldie doesn't have eyes. I've even been asked if Goldie can see shadows because she often appears to get around so well!! (And, of course, the answer is no. No eyes, no sight!)

So, I hope to do Goldie justice by telling her story. As she is sitting on the couch in the same room, I'm typing away on the keyboard.

In a few minutes, she'll take her walk as she does every day. She'll eat her meals as she does every day. And she'll play with her toys, as yes, she does every day.

Before Goldie, I may have never adopted a blind dog. Now my perception has drastically changed. I would indeed adopt an already blind dog! There's nothing to be afraid of! Nothing.

Blind dogs can thrive. Blind dogs can have fun. And most importantly, blind dogs can LIVE!

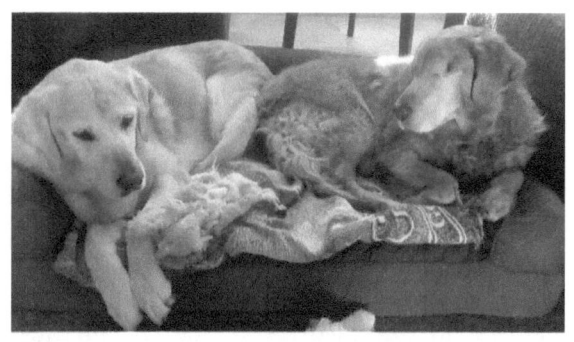

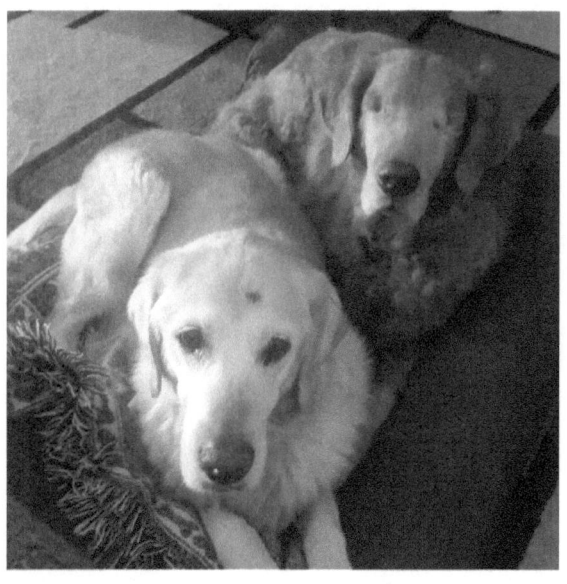

Chapter 1-Glaucoma

I look into the eyes of my dog, or at their face, or see a picture of a dog I've never met. Instantly, I see love, trust, truth, innocence, curiosity, and hope... and my heart skips a beat.

There's no guesswork. No games, no lies. They speak not one word of our language, yet convey their very thoughts to us and understand what we say to them. They know our moods before we do, and strive to cheer us up. They are the best counselors, friends and companions, and don't have room for judgment, head games or deceit. What you'll get is only pure, unfiltered love. If you still have to ask "why dogs?" perhaps you'll never understand.

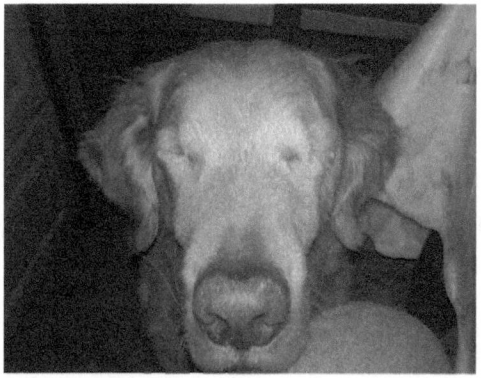

Dogs hold the key to our hearts. They know just how to give us that certain look, or perk up their ears, or wag their tail and wiggle their body in an endearing way that makes us dog lovers drop what we're doing and lean in for a hug.

The love we receive from a dog is unprecedented. Never is there judgment, or criticism. There is no anger or game playing. With dogs, what you see is what you get. Their emotions are visible, and their body language reveals all. You always know where you stand when in the company of dogs. Or perhaps, you know where you sit or lay, depending on wherever your pooch is! The old term we've all heard over and over again rings true. Like the perfect combination of emotion-enhancing medicine, dogs administer endless doses of unconditional love.

Perhaps that is why we try to do our very best to spoil them, lavishing them with everything they deserve. We want to make sure they are happy, comfortable, well-fed, entertained and of course, healthy.

The feeding part is easy. Simply fill their bowls and announce that it's meal time. And it takes nothing to get them comfortable. A cushioned bed or a spot right next to you is all they require.

Sometimes, however, there are certain things we can't regulate. Fate has already predetermined their destiny, and their medical issues are way beyond our control.

As with any animal, dogs can suffer a wide variety of ailments. The symptoms can vary, and some are easier to resolve than others. Sadly, some have no resolution. Having lived with many dogs throughout my lifetime, I've seen many illnesses, but I had never come across a disease of the eyes, especially a dog with glaucoma.

Glaucoma can affect dogs of all ages, during any stage of their precious life. Although certain breeds are more susceptible to glaucoma, it can affect all breeds.

It is a disease that puts tremendous pressure on the eye. This pressure causes eyes not to have sufficient fluid drainage, thus, affects the optic nerve.

Unfortunately, most dogs diagnosed with glaucoma will eventually become blind.

While the symptoms may be obvious to doctors, for someone who has never become acquainted with this condition, it may seem like an allergy or eye-infection.

The symptoms can vary. Some dogs have all the symptoms, and some only possess some. At least at first. Noticeable symptoms consist of a cloudy eye, excessive blinking, redness, and enlargement of the eyeball.

Some dogs may show their discomfort by refusing to eat or play. Some may be lethargic. When the eye pressures are high, the pain is similar to a severe migraine.

I'm able to recite these facts now, however, rewind a few years, and I knew nothing at all about the disease.

That is until I adopted Goldie.

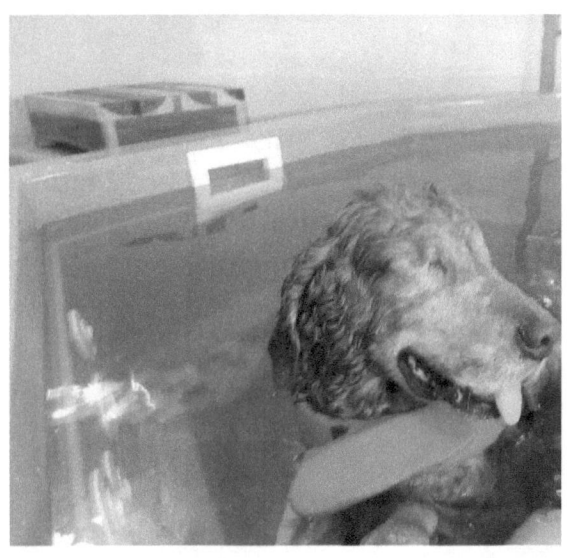

\

Chapter 2-The Search Begins

We rely on our senses to live, while dogs rely on the scents to make sense. Without speaking a word, or delving into the history of someone they have only just met, they immediately know the difference between friend or foe. I fully trust in the judgment of a dog and respect their decisions wholeheartedly.

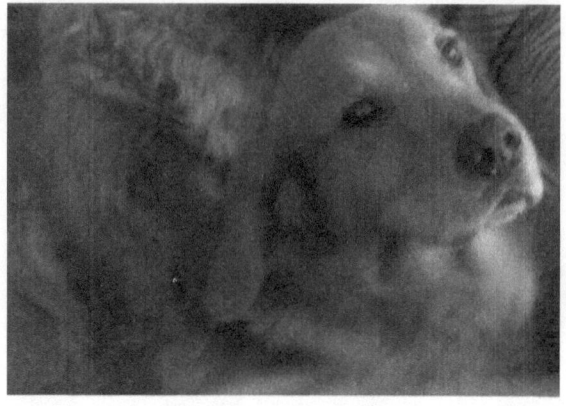

I was living on Long Island, New York at the time. Normally, I've had two to three dogs at a time, but during this period, I only had one. His name was Duke.

Duke was a handsome, regal golden retriever. Sweet as could be with humans, he took pride in his status when meeting other dogs.

Or at least he took pride in the status he thrived for, but had yet to achieve!

See, Duke always competed for alpha status. When he had come into my home years before, he had Lyme disease. The first couple of months with him were spent trying to nurse him back to health. He could barely walk and didn't have an appetite. It was a long struggle, but thankfully, he pulled through and finally started walking and regained his golden retriever appetite!

I had already owned two other resident dogs at the time, Brandi and Toffee. Both were super friendly. While Duke was sick, he barely interacted with them as he didn't have the energy.

Toffee would frequently lay next to him and kiss him, to which he responded with a weak growl. She didn't relent and eventually, either too weak to argue or perhaps he just realized she was persistent, he gave in and let her kiss him. She was happy, and he appeared content.

After Duke fully recovered, however, he tried his very best to establish alpha status with Brandi.

Brandi was an agile, healthy, golden retriever who had proudly and successfully held alpha status for years. Not only with my dogs, but with dogs she met at the park or on the street. She earned her respect, and other dogs never seemed to mind. In fact, they were happy to see her. She was always the leader of the group and kept everyone in line.

When new dogs were introduced, either to visit or to live with us, my job was easy. It was Brandi who did all the work!

Brandi trained them and showed them the ropes with nothing more than a slight nudge here and a little growl there. She was always in control, never escalating a doggy argument beyond that growl.

So, when Duke attempted to take rise to the top of the hierarchy, she laughed in his furry face the best way dogs know how, and she gently, but firmly put him in his place.

It didn't happen overnight, as Duke had to try two or three times before he realized he wasn't any match for Brandi who was much smaller than himself!

He tried everything from stealing her toys to trying to "help" her eat her food. Neither was in his best interest!

Once he realized she was serious and not budging, he obliged and accepted his position with grace. He stuck to eating only out of his food bowls and didn't dare try to steal a toy Brandi had in her possession.

During their time together, Brandi, Toffee, and Duke lived harmoniously together and were the utmost best of friends. Each had their quirks, and all of them respected the other.

They ate together, played together and slept together without incident. The trio was truly a pack. All were special in their own way.

Duke and Brandi loved toys, and while Brandi gravitated toward the toys that were almost the same size as her, Duke was happy with toys he could easily manage.

Toffee carried one special toy around—and kept this toy for all the years of her life. She sometimes explored new stuffed animals or examined new gifts, but always ventured back to her green, plastic squeaky toy shaped like a dog. This toy was hers, and Brandi and Duke didn't try to pass it off as their own.

It was almost as if they understood and respected the importance of this toy to Toffee.

Truly a group of best friends who never were far from one another.

After Toffee passed away suddenly from a mal seizure and then six months later, Brandi passed away from hemangiosarcoma, Duke was lonely.

It was true now that he was the king of the castle, as he was the only dog. I can only imagine he would have proudly worn a crown while sitting atop his thrown, but he settled for having his choice of stuffed animals instead!

Even though he had loved his sisters dearly, his intentions upon meeting dogs in the street were questionable. I had to be cautious with Duke as he wouldn't play nicely with others at first, so adopting a new dog would be a trying experience.

While not a vicious dog, he was just difficult in the "beginning" stages of making new friends. Once he made friends, he was friends for life. Docile and even submissive.

Judging by the way he followed me everywhere after Brandi passed away, it was apparent he was lonely. He went from living with his two sisters to having only me.

I knew I had to adopt a friend for him, and quite honestly, I missed having two additional dogs as well!

Each day, I sifted through the rescue sites in search of a golden retriever who needed a home.

Surprisingly, there were not many available. There were puppies, however, I did not think that would be a good fit for Duke. While still energetic, Duke was approaching his 12th birthday. He needed a dog somewhat close to his age.

The months went on, and finally, I saw one whom I thought would be the perfect match.

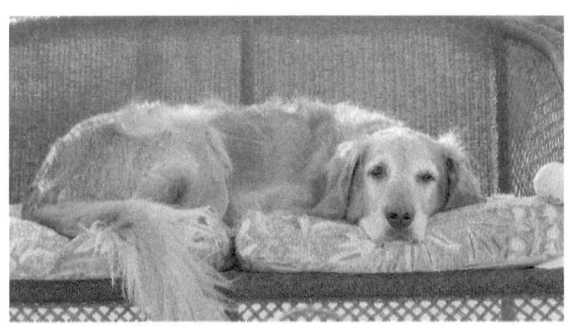

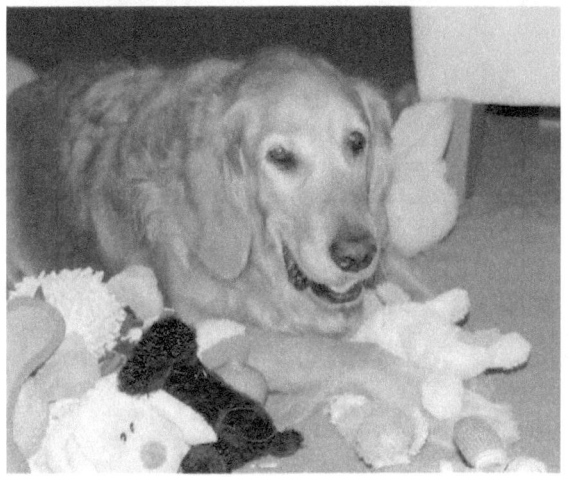

Chapter 3~GOLDIE!

It has been said that good things are worth waiting for. There are no truer words. Indeed, the best things in life are worth the wait.

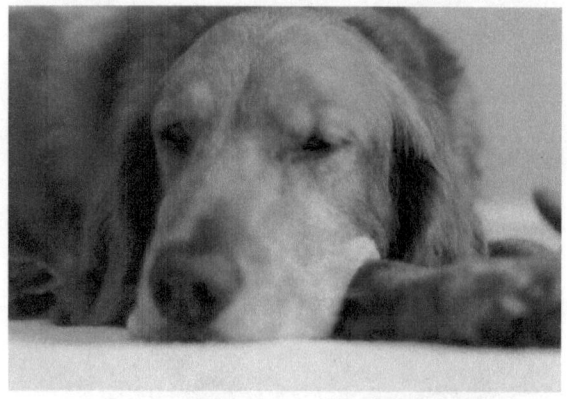

In my search for another dog, I began to grow a little impatient. Duke and I both had oodles of love to give to a dog in need, but most were younger, so we waited.

When I finally saw the ad, I grew hopeful. A red-haired golden, she was listed as being approximately eight years old and was friendly with other dogs. The ad said her foster parent loved her and she was a respectful house guest with perfect manners. I couldn't wait to meet her.

After going through the necessary channels, I spoke with the rescue coordinator.

She requested a house visit, as most rescue groups do, and came by a few days later.

During a home visit, certain things are checked for such as environment, gated yards and sleeping conditions for the dog, along with seeing if there are children in the home, other pets, etc. The coordinator will judge if the household is a good fit and decide based on what they find.

Since Duke slept in a bed, and was allowed on the furniture and ran freely in my fenced yard with his pick of numerous toys, I was confident my house would be approved, however, I was still quite nervous! Luckily, all was approved, and we were onto step two!

The next step was introducing the two dogs and observing how they interacted with each other.

On a Saturday afternoon, the dog-rescue coordinator called me and set up a time to meet at the park with Duke and Goldie.

Slightly nervous about how Duke would behave, I gave him a little lecture on the way there, and his ears perked up as he listened intently, or at least placated me and pretended to pay attention!

Once we pulled into the parking lot, he saw Goldie walking around and didn't have much of a reaction. This was a good sign.

I always noticed with Duke, that if he didn't show much interest in a dog, then he would get along with them instantly.

It was now time to test that theory. I helped him out of the car and walked him over to Goldie and introduced myself to Goldie's foster mom.

The moment I saw Goldie, I fell in love instantly. She was smaller (and wider) than most goldens I've had and walked through the park as if she didn't have a care in the world.

Now it was Duke's turn to make his judgment call. This was the moment for which I had been waiting.

Ready for anything, I loosely held onto his leash as I didn't' want him to sense any of my anxiety.

Much to my chagrin, Duke strolled over to Goldie. They both sniffed each other in the proper dog manner, then showed no interest and sniffed the grass. Both walked around the park together like they had been old high school buddies, on a leisurely outing.

All of the worry and anxiety about how Duke would react was for naught! Not one growl, not one display of discomfort or fear and not one hint of aggression from either. Whew!

It is these moments that I only wish I had captured on camera because the meeting was lovely!

It was a BEAUTIFUL match!

Within minutes Duke had a sister, and I had a new fur-baby!

She was amazing. I watched as she stood up and hugged her foster mom goodbye. A vision that brought tears to my eyes. She was the most loving and sweet dog. My only hope was that she would develop that same bond with Duke and I.

From the start, Duke and Goldie were best of friends, following each other everywhere. Goldie fit right in, ate in her designated food bowl, slept on her side of the bed, followed the rules and didn't cause any problems whatsoever.

The initial ad about her was completely accurate. Goldie was the perfect house guest and had impeccable manners!

I watched the two dogs closely as I always do when introducing a new dog into the house and they got along famously. Within days, they only had one minor argument about a toy, which was just Goldie growling at Duke for taking it, but it was enough to determine their status.

Goldie was the new alpha. She accepted her role without flaunting it, and Duke graciously accepted his without complaint. Poor Duke, as much as he vied to be alpha, it was just never meant to be! But he loved Goldie, and that was all that mattered.

She was a charm. On our first walk together, she stopped mid-way, turned and looked up at me, her brown eyes wide and intense. I wasn't quite sure why she had stopped, but she soon let me know.

Looking straight into my eyes, she then jumped up, giving me the biggest, most lovable hug.

She held on tightly for a few moments.

It was the kind of hug where her paws wrapped as far around my waist as far as they could go and she nestled her head against my stomach, welcoming my hug in return.

I have to say; it took my breath away. I felt "accepted" and special that this dog only knew me a few hours and gave me the same hug she gave her foster mom. I felt as if she now recognized me as her new mom and Duke as her new brother.

Then we walked a little more, met a boy in the street, and then…she looked up at him with the same loving look, and yes, she hugged him too.

And, you guessed it. A few more blocks, another person, and she hugged them as well. She couldn't walk past a person without hugging them. Although she initially feared some men, she hugged almost everyone she met!

In the human equivalent, it was as if she was introducing herself to the new neighborhood and greeting each neighbor with love instead of a tray of baked goods!

While my initial feeling of being "accepted" dwindled just a little, it was replaced with a heartwarming sensation that this little dog — who had been moved from wherever she started out, to a shelter, to foster-care to her new home —had enough love and trust in her heart to make everyone she met feel special and loved.

And her hugs weren't just a quick hello. They were warm and gentle as she nestled her head in and grabbed on tight, just savoring the attention from the people she met. The type of hug that could lift anyone's mood.

Living with Goldie was a blessing. She made Duke happy, and I couldn't be prouder of them both.

They often slept right next to each other, legs overlapping each other's legs, heads on each other's back. There were moments I'd simply sit in silence and watch them, amazed by their endearing friendship.

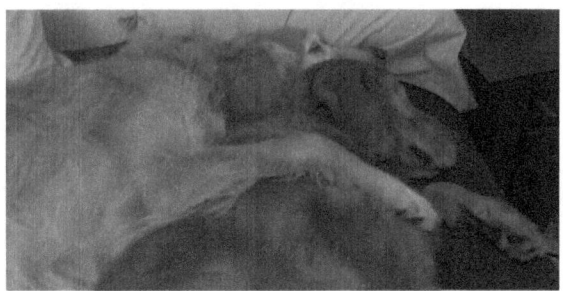

Chapter 4-Facing the Truth

Decisions. The real ones. The ones that break your heart and challenge your soul. The ones that tear at your heartstrings and have you pacing in circles frantically searching for an easier way.

Those are the ones that matter.

The right decision is typically the hardest, but lead with your heart and be the most altruistic you can be. Tears may follow, as may anger and despair. But in the long run, you'll know you did the right thing. You'll know you did all you can do and the only decision left to make was the one you hoped and prayed to avoid.

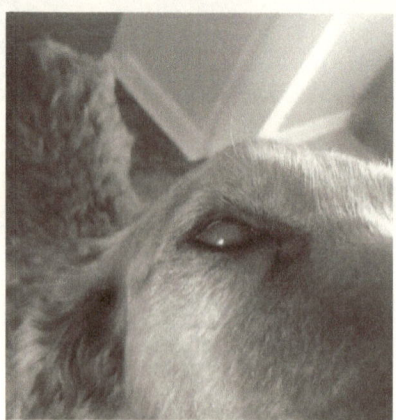

The months went by and around the holidays, in December 2015, Goldie's eye began tearing.

I've seen it before with my previous dogs, and usually, the cause was allergies, so I wanted to wait a couple of days before taking her to the vet.

I changed my mind after the second day as it seemed to be getting worse. I thought it best to get it checked out, just in case there was an infection or at the very least to ease her discomfort, if any.

The veterinarian told me her eye was just cloudy and just gave me eye drops to put in a few times per day. I asked him if it was cataracts, or glaucoma (not knowing anything about either) and he assured me she was totally fine.

Just allergies.

I believed him, after all, he was a licensed doctor. He should know, right? Wrong!

It was another week before I grew very concerned as the drops were not helping. In fact, her eye was tearing more. My instincts told me to see another veterinarian, and I'm thankful that I did.

When I first adopted Goldie, her eye had been cloudy already. She didn't show any signs of pain, however, so it was only when her cloudy eye also began tearing that the symptoms started to reveal themselves.

At first glance at the cloudy eye, the new veterinarian looked very concerned.

I told them what the first vet had told me and he shook his head. "I don't want to alarm you, but I think she might have glaucoma. We will need to run some tests."

Again, not knowing anything about this disease, I didn't understand the grim look.

The doctor put a few drops in Goldie's eyes and then took an instrument to measure the pressure in her eyes.

Once again, he gave me a sympathetic look and said, without a hint of doubt in his voice. "I'm very sorry to tell you this, but Goldie's eye pressure is 35."

I can only imagine the perplexed expression I had on my face because I still didn't know what he meant! So, heart racing, having no idea what was going on with Goldie, I asked questions.

The doctor then gave me the rundown on this disease. A rundown I wasn't quite prepared for.

He informed me that glaucoma is a very painful disease, and the higher the eye pressure, the more painful it is. A normal pressure for dogs is between zero and twenty.

Goldie's eye pressure was 35.

This is the equivalent of an unbearable migraine headache. She was, indeed, in a lot of pain.

He strongly suggested I see an ophthalmologist immediately and so the next day, off we went.

I had no idea what Goldie was going through. I figured, stronger eye drops and perhaps some medication and Goldie would be on her way to recovery.

Never in my life had I been so completely wrong!

The eye-specialist ran her own series of tests and came back wearing that same grim look.

Not only did Goldie have glaucoma, but she also had fibrin clots, golden retriever uveitis, and her vision was failing in her right eye, if there was any vision at all. The doctor thought Goldie might even be blind in the right eye!

When she lifted Goldie's eyelid, she shone a light inside. Once again I wasn't prepared to see what lingered inside.

The doctor pointed out how red and inflamed it was. While not visible without this light, it became painfully apparent that what was going on with Goldie's eyes was indeed a serious condition.

Good old eye drops weren't doing a darn thing for Goldie.

It was about this point that my heart broke. I agonized. The endless thoughts going through my mind were of such regret and frustration. Even though I had never even looked up symptoms of glaucoma, I felt I should have somehow known about this disease. I should have somehow been able to prevent this.

The doctor assured me that since her eye was already in the progressive stages when I adopted Goldie, there would have been nothing I could have done to prevent glaucoma. However, it WAS time to take action.

I had this dog for months and didn't have a clue that she was suffering! What did this all mean? Can't this be cured? There's got to be SOMETHING we can do!

And there was. But I didn't like the answer.

I downright hated the answer.

If there was ever an answer I could despise, this was the one. Like a child, I wanted to throw a temper tantrum and prove this doctor was wrong, or evil, or losing her mind or…all of the above!

This vet's strong suggestion was to remove the eye. While the other eye still had vision and the pressure was low, she even suggested removing both as it was only a matter of time.

I will admit that at this point, I was fuming. I thought it was simply a way for the surgeon to make money and that medicines would have to help. Perhaps the vision could never be restored, but certainly, the medications could bring the pressures down, prevent any more damage!

So, I told her I would think about it and asked for alternatives. She did say I could try the medications. Three different drops, spread out three times per day each, five minutes apart, along with Rimadyl for the pain.

Anything was better than removing this poor dog's eye, so that was the route I took. Before I left the vet's office, however, she pulled me aside and gently told me that surgery would most likely have to happen. She advised me she had been doing this for years and never saw the medications work long-term.

Still secretly angry, I acknowledged her advice and went home, determined to prove her wrong.

After getting Goldie settled, I ran to my computer and conducted as much research as possible on this disease. Desperately scrolling through every site, looking for one glimpse of hope, my anger slowly dissipated and quickly turned into sorrow.

Everything the veterinarian had told me was right there in front of me. It was nearly inevitable that Goldie would have to have her eye enucleated.

Still desperately clinging onto hope like Velcro to cloth, I tried the medications on her. And they worked. I grew hopeful.

But, again as the vet advised, they only worked for three months before the pressure built up again. Goldie got checkups every week, and by March, the medicines stopped working altogether. She had lost full sight in her right eye.

When faced with the type of situation that requires you to make a difficult decision, all sorts of thoughts go through your mind. You are your dog's caregiver, and as such, you're supposed to put the dog's needs before your own.

During this time, I had questions volleying back and forth, like a ball in my own personal tennis match.

First, the words of the doctor resonated. "The eyes need to be removed." "Goldie is in pain." "She might not even have vision."

Those were the phrases I kept repeating to myself. Then, I questioned them. "Do they really need to be removed?" "Is she REALLY in pain? Sometimes it doesn't seem like it." "She can see, can't she?"

A heavy onset of anxiety and negativity overwhelmed me. First and foremost, anesthesia while normally safe is not always foolproof. People and animals HAVE died from it. As with any surgery, there CAN be complications. What if Goldie didn't make it? What if she had a bad reaction?

What if she did make it through surgery, but afterward, she was miserable? What if she couldn't adjust to being blind? Would I have just "ruined" my dog's life? Would she still be able to go on walks, eat without any issues, move around the house?

Then there were the silly questions, but at the time, seemed so relevant. Would Goldie still have facial expressions? Would I be able to determine if she was awake or asleep? Would she be depressed? Would I? Was I strong enough to train a blind dog? Would I learn how to train her? Could I help her?

That was perhaps one of my biggest concerns. I had never owned a blind dog before. I had no idea what to expect. What if I couldn't lead her in the right direction? What if I wasn't able to determine what she wanted? Would she still have the same personality? Would I know if she was uncomfortable?

At the time I felt there was such relevance in those questions and I had answers for none of them.

Still, I had to put my concerns to the side and face them at a later date. At that moment, I had to focus on Goldie and Goldie only.

For some facing a similar situation, other questions may arise, such as which doctor should perform the surgery, your primary veterinarian or a doctor that specializes in ophthalmology.

For me, I didn't really have a choice as my primary veterinarian did not perform that type of surgery. However, had I been given the option, I believe I still would have chosen the ophthalmologist.

For one, an experienced ophthalmologist has seen this type of disease (and others like it) numerous times. The surgeon I had used had been a doctor for over twenty years. She performed enucleations thousands of times. With any surgery, there is always the risk of complications, and I felt comfortable knowing that this doctor knew the procedure inside and out and would recognize and be able to rectify a complication should one arise.

Also, when the surgeon visibly noticed my uneasiness about the entire surgery, she said one thing that put my mind at ease. The gist of what she said was this: "If for nothing else, trust in me in a selfish way. I rely on my job to pay my bills, and I rely on your happiness to keep my job. I studied for years to get to where I am now and have invested a lot of time and money to be a surgeon. I don't want to do anything to risk that, so, I'm going to do everything I can to make sure your dog has both a successful surgery and a healthy recovery."

It was those very words that gave me the comfort I needed. She was right. She was a reputable surgeon and would put her all into making sure Goldie had the most successful surgery possible. This meant bloodwork beforehand and constant monitoring during and after surgery.

Her staff of veterinary technicians and assistants were fabulous with Goldie, showing her oodles of attention and love. They assured me I could call any time if I think of additional questions and during each time that I had to bring Goldie in for a spike or checkup, the staff went above and beyond in accommodating me. I felt she would be in good hands should I go through with the surgery.

I believe your instincts kick in when facing a major decision like this. You have to feel that not only the surgeon but the staff has your dog's best interests at heart.

While there is nothing you can do to ease your anxiety if your pet goes through surgery, knowing that they are in a caring facility makes all of the difference.

That being said, after many sleepless nights, I was finally able to think it through. The harsh logic had prevailed, and here it was.

Without surgery, Goldie would live the rest of her days in excruciating pain and to top things off; it would only get worse. It was questionable if she could even see in her current state. There was no hope for her to get better. That would be the life she'd lead.

Just those thoughts alone propelled me forward into thinking logically.

Yes, she could die under surgery. Yes, she could be miserable AFTER surgery.

Since I never want to allow my dogs to suffer, I couldn't let Goldie live her life as she was. I couldn't wake up to her each morning to find she was in pain, every hour of every day. That just wasn't fair.

The blatant truth was if any of my dogs had a painful condition that could not be managed with medications, I would be facing the dreadful choice of euthanasia.

There were only three decisions to choose from, and none of them were good ones. One, let her live a life in pain. Two, have an otherwise very healthy dog euthanized. Three, opt for the surgery and have the utmost faith that everything would work out for the best.

As I was trying to make this decision, I even flew back to Las Vegas for work for a few days, and while there, visited my old veterinarian to get his advice! My goal was to talk to anyone and everyone who had experience with this disease.

After agonizing for days, beating myself up with self-doubt, questioning the validity of Goldie's condition and reading as much as I could on this disease, I finally made a choice.

I chose option three.

I also rationalized with myself that while blindness wasn't going to be a picnic for Goldie, that it was a little different for dogs. Dogs don't have to drive, or read, or work. They could function better than we think they can. They have us humans to care for them.

It was the only logic I could conjure up, and I had to believe in Goldie and…believe in myself, and the surgeon!

With that, my decision was made. Goldie would get the surgery, and I would pray and hope that there would be no complications.

I would pray some more that she wouldn't hate me for deciding that for her.

And I hoped upon hope that once her surgical site healed, that she would be able to enjoy life still. That she would still be Goldie. And that blindness didn't conquer her. I had hoped that Goldie, somehow, some way, would conquer her disability and move forward.

Yes, it would be a different life, but I had to think positive and do my very best to make her new life a good one and one yes, without eyes, but also a life without pain.

Through tears, I agreed to the surgery, and it was scheduled for the end of the week.

I knew it was pointless to let her suffer. She couldn't see out of the affected eye. It was doing her more harm than good.

I had no idea how quickly, however, she would then lose her sight in the other eye.

It was all too sudden.

Knowing she would be getting surgery in a few days, I tried to make each day extra special until then.

We had a great day, went on a walk and played a little. After a few hours, she laid down for a nap, and I went into the other room to do some work.

A few hours later, it was Goldie and Duke's favorite time of day—dinner!

I called her to eat, and she didn't come. With Goldie, she ALWAYS listened when called.

Assuming she didn't hear me, or perhaps she was in a really deep sleep, I went to get her.

There she was, standing on the bed, a terrified look on her face. Her left "good" eye was now cloudy and enlarged. I knew instantly she couldn't see out of the left eye now too but had no idea why!

Dropping everything, I started to carry her down the stairs. With a sixty-pound Goldie in my arms, I fell on the stairs! Don't worry; Goldie didn't fall out of my arms. I made sure of that, so I was the only one who got hurt!

Once we were safely down the fourteen steps, I got up, brushed myself off, ignored the pain in my own back and got Goldie steady on her feet. I then let her walk on a leash to the door and then to the car. Frantic and worried, I rushed her to the eye specialist.

Again, more tests were run, and the doctor explained Goldie had what's called a spike. This means the pressure in the "good eye" rose to above 35. She gave Goldie glycerin and thankfully, the vision returned.

Crisis averted.

Temporarily.

Goldie had another spike the day after the first one. While it's not proven if glaucoma progression in each eye is independent of the other, the consensus was that the bad eye could have possibly caused the "good" eye to have these spikes.

We could no longer wait until the end of the week to do surgery. Time was working against us. The glycerin didn't work quite as well the second time, and the pressures were rising.

I scheduled emergency surgery for the next day, which happened to be St. Patrick's Day of 2016. Goldie had to stay overnight to be monitored.

During all of this, the previous weeks, Duke had been having tests of his own. A large growth on his mouth was suspected to be melanoma. Over the weeks leading up to this, he had X-rays and ultrasounds at this same facility, with an oncology specialist.

Sadly, the day that Goldie went in for surgery wasn't a good day at all. Unfortunately, on this same day after dropping Goldie off, I had been taken into a separate room with Duke. The oncologist had that sympathetic look, and I didn't need him to say another word.

But, he did.

I was told Duke had melanoma that had metastasized to his lungs. The doctor told me there was nothing we can do as the cancer was too far advanced.

I then asked that dreadful question. I already knew the response wouldn't be good. I already knew my heart was about to get broken. I already knew that the news I was about to hear would crush me, but still, I had to ask. "How long does he have?"

The pursed lips, the sympathetic look. I knew it all too well.

There was no way to sugar coat this. The doctor must have given this news to pet owners dozens of times, but I could see him struggle as he was about to tell me the horrid truth. And then he did.

The prognosis was dire. My sweet angel Duke would only have two to three months to live.

I sat in utter disbelief. I kneeled on the cement floor and took Duke in my arms. As I hugged him tightly, the tears poured down my face and onto his beautiful golden fur. It felt like the ground was moving, but I think it was my sobbing that seemed to have shaken the room.

This couldn't be happening. I was hoping the news would be better. I was praying that the growth on Duke's mouth was just a lipoma, a simple growth, or a minor annoyance.

But that was not the case.

I wanted to close my eyes and open them, hoping this was all a horrible nightmare. My heart pounded on my chest as the realization kicked in.

I couldn't bear to lose Duke.

Trying to make sound decisions was extremely difficult, and I had to try my best to put my emotions aside and make sure both dogs were to live as comfortably as they could.

To look at Duke during this time, one would never know he was sick, aside from a growth on the side of this mouth. The best I could do was keep a close watch on him and watch for any changes in his breathing.

My world was spinning upside down. Duke— who was my shadow and one of the sweetest, most loyal dogs— had only months left. Duke, who came to me only a few years ago suffering from Lyme disease for months until he recovered. Duke was finally able to walk again, and play and enjoy life…and was now getting his life stolen from him. And all at this same time, Goldie was going through her challenge.

Leaving her at the vet's office overnight was the last thing I had wanted to do. I wanted to stay with her, but I knew that wasn't feasible.

To say I was terrified is an understatement, but I had to do what was best for Goldie. Living with that much pain is no way to live, and I had to do whatever I could to make her comfortable. I just hoped she would forgive me!

If my memory serves me correctly, I had the phone in one hand waiting to hear from the surgeon and hugged Duke with the other hand for most of the day.

I anxiously awaited the call from the surgeon. Finally, in the afternoon, she called and said Goldie did wonderfully. They did let me know that due to the after-effects of anesthesia, she was a bit uneasy, so they gave her a sedative to calm her down.

Hearing about Goldie's uneasiness upset me, but the doctor explained why. When the anesthesia begins to wear off, some dogs can experience a sort of a state of confusion or similar effects to a hangover. Some may cry and pace, as Goldie did. Once they gave her a sedative, she relaxed and slept.

They advised that I didn't see her as she was sleeping comfortably, but that I could pick her up the next day. I wanted nothing more than to see her, but I took their advice, trying to keep Goldie's best interests in mind.

The following morning, I called the vet's office. I wouldn't be able to pick her up before 9, but they advised me I could call any time before then for a status update.

I called at 5 A.M, the moment I opened my eyes. The vet tech said she was doing wonderfully. They let me know she went potty outside and ate her breakfast.

Even though I heard what they told me, I knew I wouldn't feel better until I saw for myself.

I arrived at the vet's office before 9 and waited patiently until I would be allowed to see her and take her home.

Not knowing what to expect. I thought Goldie would be sad and lethargic. It was still questionable on whether the remaining eye had any vision or not.

I waited until the vet tech brought me in the back room.

A few moments later, I heard the sound I recognized so well—Goldie shuffling through the halls.

Before I had even seen her, I heard her "happy" cry that she does when she's excited to see people.

She ran to me, dragging the vet tech behind her. And as soon as I did see HER, she jumped up and…gave me her famous warm, gentle, forgiving, sweet hug.

Chapter 5-Home Sweet Homecoming

We all have weaknesses, and either visible disabilities or simply things we can't do. You can choose to dwell on the negative, or be grateful for the positive and put your energies into forming a celebration around your successes.

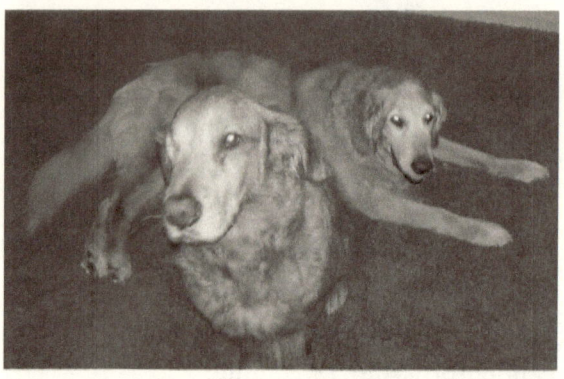

That hug. That miraculous hug from a dog that, like a magic wand, sprinkles the sensation of admiration throughout. It's the kind of unforgettable hug that bridges the gap between canine and human. The heartfelt one that dismisses any differences and demonstrates the tightest bond of love, friendship, respect, and companionship. It's that meaningful hug that can get you through the toughest of days, and warm one's heart to the greatest extent.

She knew I was there. I had to assume she could see out of the remaining eye. How else would she have been able to run toward me, find me without effort and jump up and hug me?

She had to have vision!

The vet could not confirm or deny if Goldie had vision or not. It was difficult to determine, because when they had Goldie follow their finger as they moved it back and forth, Goldie moved her head along with it. Dogs have a keen sense of smell, so she could have either followed the vet's finger through scent or by sight. And, oddly enough, it seemed like Goldie COULD see. We didn't know.

After surgery, while Goldie was physically ok, albeit a little tired, the doctor pointed out that her eyes were swollen. And indeed, they were. At first glance, I didn't think they would heal. However, the doctor assured me that it was perfectly normal.

As with any surgical site, I was prepared to observe her stitches and scar each day and make sure there was no oozing or newfound redness.

I had taken pictures of her eye to make a note each day on how it was improving.

Forgive the blurriness of this picture. I deleted most of the pictures after Goldie's wound had healed, but I hope to give an idea of what to expect.

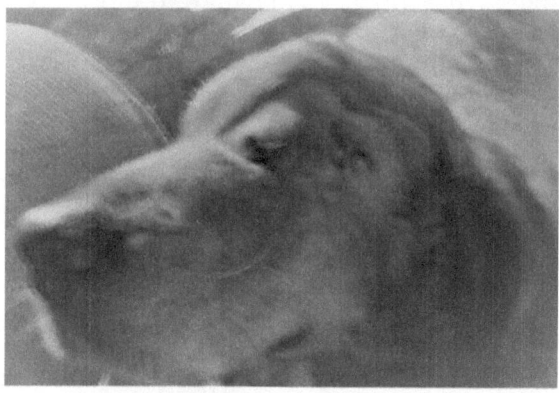

If you do find yourself in the same or similar situation, pictures help. Initially, it may seem like the wound will never heal, but with time, the swelling DOES go down an enormous amount. They will not always look as they do the day after surgery, so don't panic!

Of course, if you notice new bruising or any symptoms that resemble an infection, it's wise to call the surgeon and voice your concerns.

Checkups are a must. After the first surgery, I was told the stitches could come out in about two weeks, but it turned out to be closer to three weeks. The doctor wanted to err on the side of caution and make sure the wound was fully closed before removing any stitches.

It was a slight disappointment for Goldie as she was still wearing the cone of shame. However, she didn't complain too much, and it was better to be cautious!

One note about the cone. Dogs are determined creatures. Make sure the cone is large enough so that your pup can't stick their little feet in there and begin scratching. Goldie surprised me one day when she managed to position herself in just the right way, so she was finally able to scratch that itch!

Thankfully, I caught her in time before she did any damage. If possible, have someone with your dog during this healing process. It's difficult to do so as most of us need to leave the house at some point, but it's only for three weeks or so, and you'll be happy you were there to monitor your healing pooch!

Also, if you have other pets in the house, note how they react to your dog as she's recovering. Make sure there is no play fighting and if you find you cannot stop this from happening, it might be best to separate the animals until your pup is fully healed. One accidentally scratch could land your pup back on the operating table!!

Once she got released from the hospital, Goldie and I walked to the car and I carefully opened the car door. Again, without effort, she put her front legs up and tried to jump in on her own. Worried she might still be drowsy, I lifted her and got her settled next to my mom, who sat in the back with Goldie.

Goldie laid down on my mother's lap and didn't complain the entire way home.

Duke welcomed his sister home with open paws and stayed by her side all day, even resting his big snout inside of Goldie's cone. It was clear he had missed her!

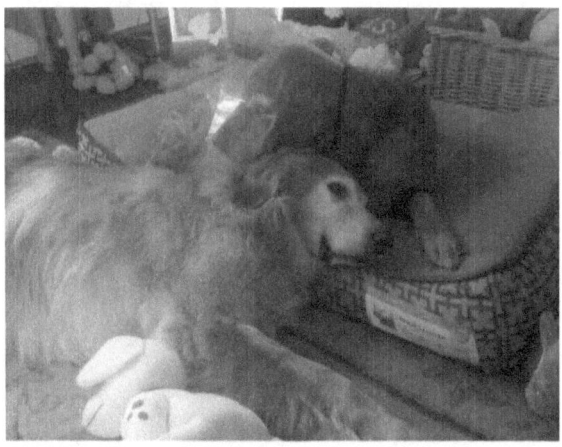

Watching them, I couldn't fathom that as fast as they had become friends, Goldie would soon lose Duke. It was nearly impossible to remain positive and upbeat, but I didn't want to reveal to them both how upset I was. I am sure that they could sense it no matter how hard I tried to hide it!

I wanted to treasure every moment with those two, and I wanted them to have each other for as long as they could.

I didn't know how Goldie would get around the house without full vision or any vision at all, but once again, she surprised me.

I had been reading up on forums about those who had experience with blind dogs of their own, and the stories varied for each. Some did well; some did not. Some didn't even seem like the blindness bothered them, and others were having a tough time with it. It's a major adjustment, so each dog reacts differently.

Certain factors contribute to Goldie's success in coping with her blindness.

For one, I have to wonder if she had been partially blind already before I had adopted her, and if so, perhaps it had been for years.

I wonder if she had previously adjusted to the reduced sight before becoming fully blind. After her surgery, she was pain-free and I believe that the pain she was suffering was more uncomfortable than the blindness itself.

Secondly, she was very healthy at the time of her surgery and had recovered fairly quickly.

Third, I strongly believe that keeping her daily routine had helped. As soon as she was able, I acted as if nothing was wrong and took her for the same walks at the same time every day and didn't treat her any differently, other than helping her when she needed help.

The first time I walked her after her surgery, I will admit, I was a bit anxious. I thought she would be scared or withdrawn. She wasn't. Since she had already walked that same route numerous times before her surgery, she didn't miss a beat! When we headed back toward the house, she turned into the driveway without me even leading her. I can't stress this enough, but their sense of smell is amazing. It is almost important as, if not just as important as their eyesight!

I know some dogs do you have trouble adjusting and the only advice I could give is this: First, make sure they are not in pain. Also, keep trying to enforce their regular routine and make sure that there are no other underlying medical issues that are affecting their progress. Of course, blindness is a big adjustment so a neurotic dog might not adjust as well. Goldie has never been neurotic or anxious, so this may have helped her succeed as well.

I often wonder if any of my previous dogs would have done well if they had gone blind. My dog Buddy (star of my book Finally Home) was neurotic when he had just to wear a cone, so I don't think he would have been able to adapt as well as Goldie had if he had ever gone blind!

Goldie maneuvered through the house fine, ate without hesitation and within two days played with her toys more than she had in months!

This isn't to say that she didn't have her moments. She didn't exactly walk a straight line, and still bumped into walls, or tripped over a step, but overall, I was amazed by her progress.

I must mention, when living with a blind dog, you can expect to receive a few accidental nudges from your pooch, and you may occasionally trip over them when they try to maneuver around unsuccessfully. Then there are the times when they move around faster than you would imagine…especially if there is food on the stove! During those times, watch out! It's almost a guarantee they will knock you over in the process!

And just a heads up, there is no such things as "rushing" when trying to lead your blind dog. Patience is key. Even though you may have them on a leash and expect them to follow, they still want to smell things on their own and feel secure in knowing where they are going! My walks with Goldie consist of Goldie sniffing every rock, every blade of grass, every scent around her. If it's windy, walks take twice as long. More scents in the air equal more time to sniff things!

Speaking from experience, leave yourself a little extra time if you are taking your blind pup for a walk or a potty break. You may be out a little while longer than anticipated!

Hopefully, if you have other resident pets in the house, they will learn patience as well.

Duke didn't seem to care when Goldie stepped on his head sometimes or bumped into him. It was like he knew she couldn't see well (if at all) and was completely supportive of her.

Seeing how much happier Goldie was after the surgery, I regretted waiting those months actually to do the surgery. I truly thought the medicines would help, and only then realized that I only prolonged the inevitable.

In the meantime, after the surgery, the doctor had prescribed pain medications, antibiotics and eye drops for Goldie's remaining eye. Hopeful that she still had sight, I wanted to do what I could to prevent any damage in her "good" eye.

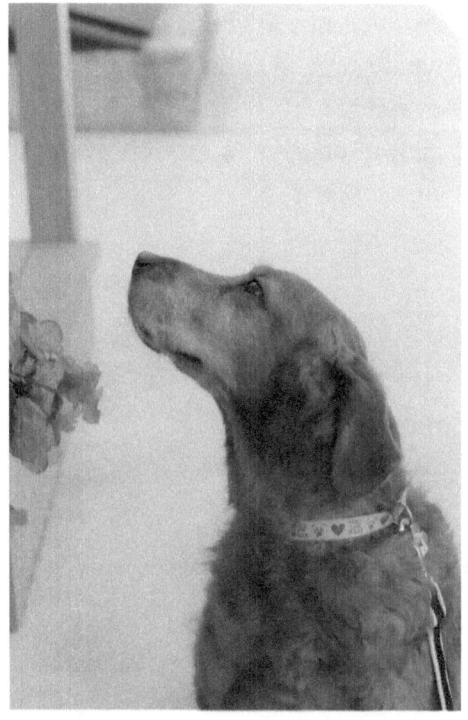

Goldie maneuvered around so well and appeared to be looking at anyone when they spoke, so I decided to wait on removing that eye. The eye pressure was in the normal range, and she did not appear to be in pain.

She went for checkups every two weeks to check on both the surgical site and the remaining eye.

She did very well, for a while. However, as bad luck would have it, a few months later, her eye pressures rose to the "painful" number, and it became apparent that she could no longer see.

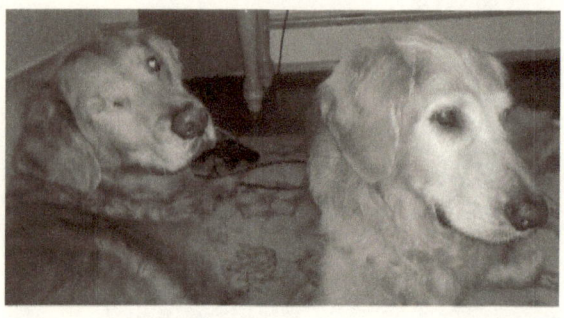

Without hesitation this time, I scheduled the second eye surgery in November of 2016. Since I had become aware of how painful this disease is, I didn't want to prolong the inevitable as I did with her first eye.

It was the best decision I could have made for her and have no regrets.

And, the good news was, Duke was still with us!

It was eight months after his original diagnosis, and he still showed no physical signs of distress, still playing, still walking around the block, still wagging his tail, eating, drinking and being a happy dog.

For Goldie's surgery, I brought Goldie to the hospital and again she had to stay overnight.

The next day, after her release from the hospital, she was happier than I had seen her been all week. Other than some discomfort for a few days, she was back to playing with her toys, going on walks, cuddling with Duke and me.

In other words, she didn't seem negatively affected by her loss of sight at all. If possible, she was happier! No more medications. No more painful eye drops. No more irritation, emergency hospital visits, and weekly checkups.

Finally, Goldie was able just to be Goldie! And, YES blind dogs without eyes DO have facial expressions. Their eye muscles still move. They let you know if they are awake or asleep and after a while, you learn to read those facial expressions just as you would by looking in their eyes.

To help her out, even if she doesn't need it, I say good morning to her every morning and goodnight to her every night. I hope that she understands the words, and realizes what time it is. I do believe it works, as she knows our daily routine.

She knows when breakfast is. She knows what time her first walk of the day is. She even goes as far as to walk into my home office at the same time each day keeping me on schedule and preventing me from being late to work! She knows when her second walk is, dinner and bedtime.

My point is regardless if they can see or not, they learn a routine. Their internal clocks are accurate, and they are smarter than we think!

My advice, (if I were ever asked) to anyone who is going through a similar ordeal is this. Don't hesitate. If the doctor strongly suggests removing the eye as it is painful to the dog, it's something you may want to consider.

It's always good to get a second opinion if that helps, however, if it is inevitable, you will save your dog a lot of pain, and not to mention, you will save yourself a lot of money.

Eye drops and pain medications and doctor visits. The price adds up. If my memory serves me correct, the monthly bill was close to $500, only to have to get the surgery anyway.

And while the surgery is expensive, it was well worth it in Goldie's case.

Chapter 6 - Coping with Blindness

So, your dog is going blind, or is blind. Don't give up hope. Don't give up patience. Your dog wouldn't give up hope on you. Nor would they give up patience. Work with them, play with them. Most of all, love them. They need you just as much as you need them.

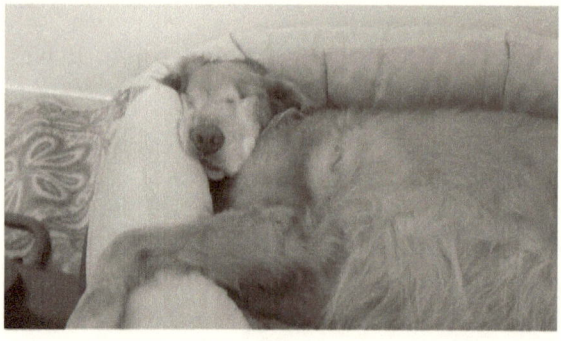

I mentioned that Goldie adapted well to her loss of sight, however, she still needed a little help. She did bump into things occasionally and was sometimes unsure of her footing. For the most part, however, she corrected herself and then found her way.

Even though emotionally, I couldn't imagine what she had endured, I always spoke to her in a positive tone as if nothing had changed.

Dogs have such keen senses and can determine our moods so easily. I never spoke to her with pity in my voice or sadness over her condition.

I felt that if I acted as if everything was okay, then she would think everything was okay. And, it seemed to work, so that is still how I speak to her till this day!

I even went as far to politely ask people who were meeting her for the first time to please don't pity her. I didn't want them leading on that something was wrong! I felt it necessary to focus on her ability rather than her disability.

Just like training any dog, positive reinforcement goes a long way. In the beginning and even still, I tried to make every accomplishment a celebration, and that seemed to help!

Since she already had known the layout of the house we lived in before going blind, she was able to get around fairly well. There were minor issues, however, when taking her out on walks on new routes, or over to my mother's house or any place for which she wasn't familiar.

It was only then that she showed any real hesitation and uncertainty in her walk. Noticing this, I did my best to help her. And believe it or not, she helped ME to help her!

She showed me certain things I would never think of by simply using her body language.

For instance, when I saw her in a tight spot, I thought I would help by lifting her and moving her to where she was trying to go. THAT was a big no-no. I quickly understood why.

While the eyes are important for a dog to see, they also rely heavily (if not more so) on their sense of smell. They know where they are just by sniffing their way around. So, when I moved her, she wasn't able to feel the floor under her feet, or smell her way to where she was going. Her body stiffened up, and her breathing became heavy.

Catching my mistake, I put her back down and put the leash on her, gently guiding her to where she wanted to go. Immediately she was at ease.

I then decided to read up on a dog's sense of smell. It is remarkable. They can get around just by scents alone. They also may smell certain things that we don't! Some dogs react to a thunderstorm before us humans can even hear the thunder. They can smell the change in the weather!

As I began to understand how important it was for Goldie to sniff her way around, I let her do so and helped only when necessary.

The house we lived in had a long set of stairs, and while I tried blocking them off, Duke would break the barricade and go up, his little sister Goldie trailing right behind. Ideally, I preferred she NOT go up the stairs when I was not home, however, I had to take measures to make sure that if by chance she got upstairs without me that she would be able to get back down.

To overcome this obstacle, we trained, using the words "step up" and "step down." Words I had never used before with her, but she understood them within a week. This made it so much easier when walking outside if we approached steps, or a curb or anything that was not straight solid ground.

In my house, she got used to the stairs; however, if we were at another location such as a park that had stairs, she would be somewhat hesitant. Usually, saying 'step up" helped, however, if she was still unsure, I took her front leg and just gently put it on the step, this way she could feel what was in front of her. She'd then climb up the rest once she finally understood there was a step in front of her.

Dogs also rely on OUR movements to guide them. Subtle movements. The kind we don't even realize that we are doing. It's incredible. Little things. For instance, when I walk Goldie and approach a curb, I instinctively now slow down. I don't consciously do it, I just do it now since I know I'm either going to have to help Goldie to give her the command to step up.

What I've noticed, however, is that when I slow down, so does she and she will automatically smell the spot in front of her. She then lifts her front paw and steps up, many times without me having to say a word!

It just goes to show you that even when you might not be training your dog, your actions DO help train them or give them guidance for any roadblocks that lie ahead!

And there are always roadblocks for which we can't help our dogs. We can help them do things on their own, and with any hope, they will map out spaces in their minds to guide them in our absence.

As an example, I didn't want always to walk Goldie on a leash inside of the house, because I believed independence would be important for her. After all, there would be times I would not be by her side, and she would have to be able to get up and move around without me.

As we trained inside the house, anytime she was about to walk into something, I'd say "Watch!" or "Watch your head" (which actually sounded like watchaed) and then she would slow down and turn another way until I said, "ok, Goldie, come on!" By just using those simple commands, she knew if I said "come" that she was heading in the right direction.

Needless to say, she still bumps into things now and then, including the backs of my legs (ouch!) but not as much as one may think!

Teaching her these commands made things much easier for both her and me.

It would only be a few months later that Goldie would be going on a road trip and seeing many new cities, states, and hotel rooms. These commands were life savers!

I'd love to take the credit and say it was me training Goldie, but with all honesty, she picked things up and listened.

She paid attention.

Goldie was the one who showed ME what she needed. Her body language revealed all. When she was "stuck," she stood still. And, although she no longer has eyes, she still has eye muscle movements. You can still read their emotions by the way they move their eyebrows that certain, telling way! It's plain to see when she requires some assistance. That's why the commands worked wonderfully. I just learned to pay attention as did she. It was a learning curve for both of us, but we made it through together.

There is such trust between Goldie and me, and I feel honored to be the one to guide her. I feel honored to have this little dog put her faith in me and feel responsible for making sure I do the best I can for her.

Chapter 7-Just a Normal Day

So, what's life like living with a blind dog? For the most part, it's not much different than living with a dog who has sight.

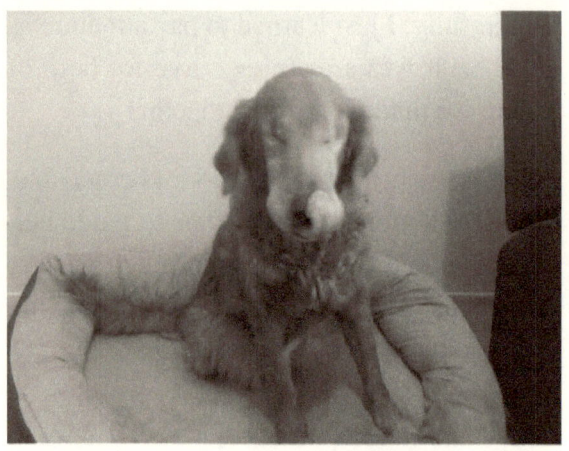

There are roadblocks, of course. Minor obstacles that may change the daily routine a little. But once you get yourself situated and find what works best for your pooch, it becomes second nature!

Those minor things are in fact minor. For instance, with all of my dogs, when they needed to go outside, I opened the door. They ran out, and I followed them. Most likely while they were doing their business, I'd be cleaning something up in the yard.

Now, I take Goldie out on a leash while Ginger runs around. If we're going to sit outside, I lead Goldie to the Chaise and she sniffs it and then jumps up. Sometimes I need to help her by lifting her back legs. This is due more to her hip dysplasia, however, than her blindness.

When we go for a car ride, I lift her into the backseat. She still tries to jump in by herself and would be able to, however, I drive an SUV and she can't jump that high. Again, it has nothing to do with her blindness! When I had a car that was low to the ground, she was still able to sniff the floorboard, put her two front paws up, find the seat and then jump with her hind legs right into her regular seat!

I do have to show her the water bowl during the day. When she's eating, however, since the bowl is right by her food bowl, she finds it on her own.

We take walks every day around the neighborhood she now knows. She still likes exploring new places and adjusts very well. She is excited to go to new parks and smell new scents!

When people come over, she still gets up to greet them. Perhaps here is where I need to help her because she gets so excited that she runs through the house and occasionally bumps into a wall here and there. So, to avoid any bumps, I try to guide her simply by running next to her. Yes, it's a funny sight!

Blind dogs get around better than we think they can. But if you find yourself with a blind dog who is having a little trouble, they do sell items you can strap to their belly or chest. It is ring shaped object that hovers over their head. The halo is one of them. It sort of blocks them from bumping into things and helps them maneuver around. It might be worth a try to see if this is something that can help your pooch get around a little easier! They can walk safely, and still eat, drink and play with this on.

Blind dogs are not much different than dogs who can see. They still love affection and still want love.

Goldie happens to love routine and truly, you can set a clock to Goldie's habits! From waking up in the morning, to her mid-morning nap, to waking up again for dinner.

There are days that I've seen her look "depressed" and normally, it's more due to the fact that she's bored. I can usually get her to be playful just by spending a little extra time with her and perhaps giving her a toy to play with or another walk.

Living with a blind dog becomes so normalized after a while that I've found myself accidentally trying to help my dog that CAN see!

Chapter 8-Duke

How do you do it? The love of your life, the one who is perhaps sitting by your side right now, the one who has been by your side since the day you brought them into your home. How do you look at them and know its time say goodbye?

How do you compensate for the loss you're about to feel and how do you actually go through with it? How do you function knowing that within a few hours you will no longer be looking at your best friend sitting by your side? Instead, most likely in a few hours you'll be clutching onto the stuffed animal that was once your best friend's favorite.

You do it because you love them enough to alleviate their suffering. You do it because as you hold their paw in your hand, you know that if they could, they would do it for you.

You do it because perhaps they didn't take their first breath with you, but their last breath will be with you holding them close, and they will know you did it because you loved them too much not to.

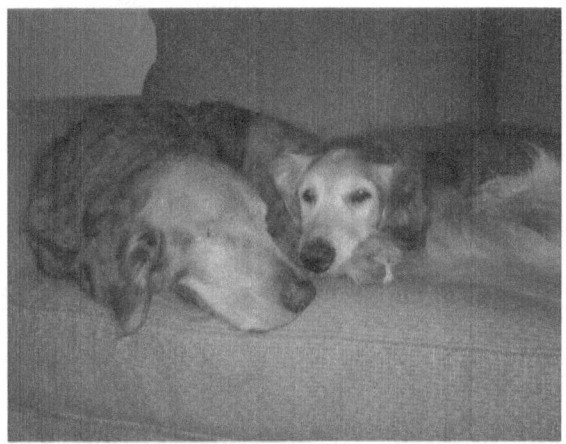

Living in NY at the time, the winters were brutal with temperatures below zero and heavy snow, but Goldie still loved the white powdery stuff no matter how cold it was and would throw her own celebration whenever she felt the heaps of that cold, white powder under her feet.

She'd roll around in it, run in it the best she could and wag her fluffy tail during her outings.

Duke was not as fond of it. Although he was intrigued by it, he did not like it as much. I had adopted Duke when I lived in Vegas, so I'm quite certain he felt the same way I did and enjoyed the heat more than the freezing cold!

He overcame his distaste for the cold, however, and during the winter months, just seemed to snuggle a bit more.

I felt blessed to have him by my side still, as he had lived much longer than had his initial prognosis. With each check-up, the doctor was amazed that the cancer in his lungs was growing at a slower rate than she originally had anticipated. That was a good thing.

Still, the cancer WAS growing.

Although I was trying to prepare for that inevitable day, I don't think there is any way you can possibly prepare yourself for loss.

You can try. You can truly cherish each day with your dog. You can make outings extra special. You can buy them extra toys. You can give them extra treats. You can lavish them with hugs and kisses. You can spend more time with them. You can pray and hope and wish upon a star that a miracle will happen and your dog will beat their illness.

But I have never been able to prepare for the day we lose them. I have never been able to conquer the heart-wrenching emotion and intense state of sadness on the day when we realize our beloved pets won't be with us anymore regardless of how much notice I had been given.

And believe me, I've tried to prepare. I've had multiple conversations with myself, repeating the same thing, trying to make sense of why our pets need to leave. But none of those self-pep talks have ever helped.

The holidays were behind us, and the stores were selling out of their Valentine's Day gifts. It was to be my first Valentine's day alone in a long time, as my divorce was finalized the previous year. I tried to put that heartache behind me and concentrate solely on my dogs.

In February, I noticed major differences with Duke. His breathing was heavy. He started slowing down, and no matter how cold it was outside, Duke was panting, and panting heavily, as if he just ran around the park a few hundred times.

Although he was still eating, I knew it was only a matter of time. Although he had lived almost a year after his diagnosis, I felt like it all happened very quickly. He seemed to have been fine one day and declined the next.

I believe dogs tell us when they are "ready" and Duke did just that.

On February 13th, he stopped eating. He didn't eat his dog food, nor his favorite foods, nor peanut butter.

Nothing.

I could see by the look in his eyes and his posture, that he was feeling horrible.

I had no choice. I refused to let my dog suffer and had to do what was best for him. These are the decisions that truly rip at your heart. Knowing they are the right decisions doesn't make it any easier.

I was going to lose my faithful boy, and there was nothing in the world I could do about it. No amount of screaming or crying could change the outcome.

When that unfortunate time comes, everything seems so surreal. There is nothing you can do to make your dog more comfortable and the realization hits.

No longer will you have your best friend there to comfort you. No longer will you see their antics, or feel their face nestled against yours. It is one of the most heart-wrenching ordeals to go through and the only one downfall of owning a pet. They leave us way too soon.

I didn't harp on my divorce like I thought I would.

Instead, I had another decision to make. Through tears, I called the vet and made the appointment for the next day, Valentine's Day of 2017.

I slept with Duke by my side and the next day, let Goldie say goodbye to him, wondering if she knew it was the last time she'd be with him. I wondered if Duke knew as well.

Still having that tiny bit of self-doubt (or maybe false hope) that comes along with making such an important decision, I asked the vet to give me her opinion, and she wholeheartedly agreed. Duke was ready to make his journey to the rainbow bridge. He was suffering.

If irony can play a part in our lives, it only seemed apropos that Duke left us on Valentine's Day. He was a huge part of my heart and will always and forever be a part of me. I do not doubt that in addition to every day when I think of him, I will think of him more every Valentine's Day and know I was never alone. I had him and am grateful I had shared a part of his life, even if it was only a few short years.

For anyone who has lost a dog, you may agree that coming home for the first time without seeing them there—wagging their tail or grabbing a toy— is one of the loneliest and heartbreaking emotions one can have. Regardless of how sick Duke had been, he always stood by the sliding glass door, a toy in his mouth and his tail wagging in excitement. When he'd see me approach, he'd run to the front door to greet me.

As I came home from the vet, the first place I looked is the sliding glass door. Of course, there was no Duke.

To top it off, seeing Goldie sniffing around for him when I walked in the door made it that much more real and final.

I couldn't mask my sadness during this time. There was no way to hide it. Goldie and I mourned together. I only hoped she wouldn't have a setback without her brother, but for a while, it appeared that she did.

One thing I always tell myself after losing a dog is that I am not getting any more dogs, the heartbreak is just too sad. I promise and vow this to myself each and every time.

However, although that might be my intention, it never works out that way.

This time, however, I was planning to move back to Las Vegas in a few months, and it wasn't logical to get another dog with the move only a few months away.

During this same time, I noticed Goldie becoming a bit withdrawn. While she was happy when out and about, or with people, she moped around the house and didn't lift a toy.

I knew then that I would have to get her a friend. It would have to be a little while.

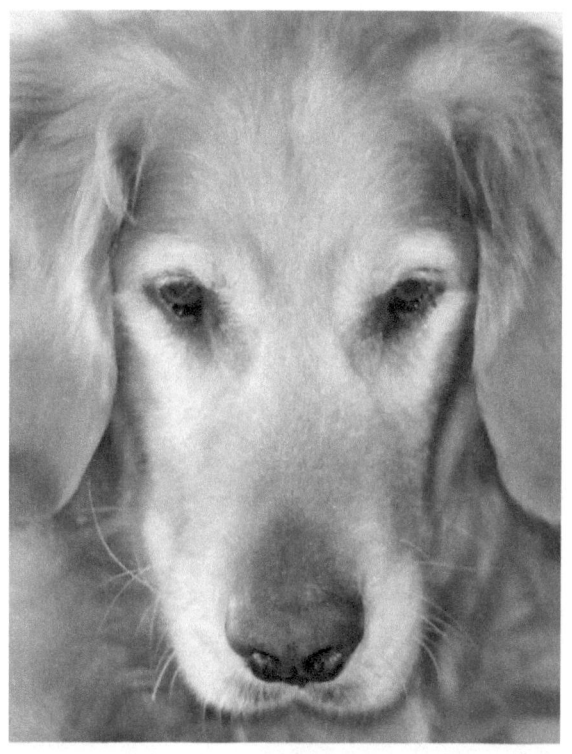

Chapter 9 -Vegas!

Life changes. At times you have to do the things that make you happiest and go to the places where you find peace. The journey, both literally and figuratively, may not be easy, but if it must be one you have to take, then take it.

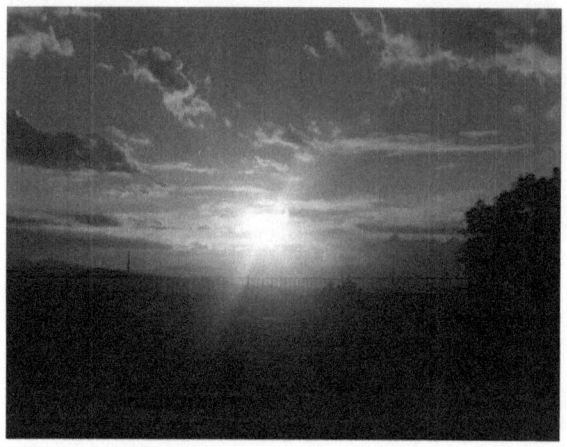

Originally, I was born and raised in New York but moved to Las Vegas in 2006. Missing family, I moved BACK to New York in 2015. The cold winters, however, were too much for me! I much prefer warmer summers and beautiful weather most of the year, so I decided to drive across the country (for hopefully that last time) back to Las Vegas.

I figured the drive would not be easy, but there was no way I was putting Goldie in cargo on an airplane, so, my niece graciously accepted my invitation for a road trip!

On the day we left, we started at 4 am. I put Goldie in her seatbelt, picked up my niece and we started our 37-hour journey!

I spent weeks preparing, trying to remember everything for the trip and making Goldie's seat as comfortable as possible as this would be the longest trip she had ever taken!

The backseat had cushions upon blankets, with pillows and plenty of space for Goldie to get up and move around while she was strapped in.

Just a side note here, doggie seatbelts are lifesavers. Thankfully during this trip, we never had to stop short and did not have any accidents, but the peace of mind knowing that Goldie wouldn't fly into the front seat was priceless.

They also help when unloading dogs from the car. Anxious dogs often want to jump out the minute the door opens, so this seatbelt restrains them until you can properly leash them and get control. There would be nothing worse than having your dog jump out and run away, especially on a busy road and/or in a state in which you were not familiar! I'm going to touch upon traveling with dogs at the end of this chapter, but in the interest of staying on course, let's get back to the trip!

As I had said, we were prepared for anything. Well, almost anything. We had one minor setback, and it was clearly my fault.

Goldie was very thirsty in the car, so I gave her a bottle of water in her bowl, which she drank. The entire bottle.

Not realizing that she had "to go" we drove an hour without stopping and, well, her comfy little bed was no longer comfy. She had a little accident and Goldie being Goldie, did not whine or give any indication that she had to go potty until it was too late!

We had to stop and improvise, so somewhere in the middle of New Jersey in the very cold weather, we threw away her plush comfy bed. Using extra blankets and pillows, we made another bed for her. She didn't seem to mind. After cleaning Goldie off, we started up again.

Just a minor setback!

As we were driving, I worried that since we would be staying in different hotel rooms across the country, that Goldie would have a tough time getting acclimated and would be scared as we entered new territory.

After all, each hotel had unique rooms with different scents for her to get used to.

She made it easy. With each hotel, we walked in with Goldie on a leash. I let her sniff around before even unloading the car. We walked around the entire room, introducing her to each couch and bed and each corner of the room.

Once that was done, Goldie was fine! Dare I say, she was even happy. I suppose we all were as, after driving fourteen-hour days it was nice to stretch out, relax and catch up on much-needed sleep!

To get our circulation moving, we all went for walks at night around the hotels and Goldie seemed to enjoy sniffing her surroundings and exploring new things.

Thank goodness for small miracles.

After four days of driving, we finally arrived at our new home.

I was excited to show Goldie where she'd be living.

Once again, I took her for a walk throughout the house and showed her the yard.

She obliged willingly without fear.

Sometimes I have to take a step back and realize dogs don't always understand what we are saying, but Goldie sure did act as if she did.

She learned the layout of the house within a day.

We walked around the neighborhood, and once she got her bearings, she even could walk up to our house without error.

I have to suppose it's because she has a great sense of smell. People have stopped me and asked, "she really can't see?" That's when I point to her eyes, and they completely get it. Nope, no possibility that she can see!!

I had briefly touched on the topic of a dog's sense of smell in a previous chapter. This is very important when getting your dog used to your house or introducing to a new house.

Since they rely on smell now that they can't see, little things we would never ordinarily think about playing a big role in a blind dog's success.

For instance, candles, scented plug-ins, potpourri, air freshener, etc. While we might never think twice about replacing one scented candle with another, a blind dog may become a little disoriented with the new smell.

What I usually do in that instance, is replace the candle and then walk my dog around the house a few times. The same route she always takes, but now with the new scent in the room. I've found it helps her get her bearings on where she is, and she soon realizes that the room didn't change, only the scent did. Surprisingly, it does not take her too long to get acclimated with the room and soon understands where she is.

Leaving shoes around or moving furniture is not helpful. Even leaving table chairs pulled out can throw a blind dog off, and as predicted, they will bump into those things that are "out of place."

In a full household, it is difficult to keep things in one place. However, there is one exercise you can do that will help you understand.

One easy way to judge what your dog is going through is to close your eyes and walk ten feet.

Seems like an easy task, right? Actually, it is a little frightening.

Now, imagine if someone left a toy in your path or a chair in a place that you weren't expecting. At best you may bump into it, but at a dog's height, hitting their head on something or tripping over an object can cause severe injury, especially if they have gained momentum and were walking quickly!

Of course, each day is a learning experience. It's learn-as-you go. Sometimes you will make mistakes, and hopefully, they can be easily resolved.

I've learned many things along the way and really hope some of these tips help if you are new at living with a blind pet.

Also, here are a few tips regarding traveling with your pet that I've learned along the way!

Over the years and after having the opportunity to share my life with many dogs, I've also taken many road trips with them. Most were enjoyable, but some could have ended up a disaster. Thankfully, the result was valuable lessons learned and never forgotten.

As a pet owner, you can try to plan for everything, but there's always one little thing you may not have thought of. I believe sharing these tiny, but potentially life-saving tidbits of information can help all of us have safe and fun travels when we bring along our pets!

One item I had never used in previous years was the doggy seatbelt. Since Goldie had gone blind, this seatbelt has proved to be a life-saver! It's very simple to use and is comfortable for your pooch. It's simply a harness that has one loop on the top of the back portion. That loop gets connected to a hook that is attached to your actual car's seatbelt. It not only prevents your dog from propelling forward should you stop short or worse, get into an accident, but it also prevents them from jumping out of the car once you have stopped and open the door to let them out! A wonderful way to prohibit your dog from getting loose and/or jumping out of the car and hurting themselves, especially if you have a truck that is high off the ground.

Next is the window lock mechanism. Dogs love to stick their heads outside the window whiffing the new scents that zip by. It's very easy for a dog to step on the button that controls the window WHILE their heads are sticking out of the window! If not caught in time, the window will keep rising resulting in a very hurt puppy, or even worse, death. Once you are comfortable with the height of the window, press that window lock button to ensure your pooch cannot raise or lower the window on their own!

Whether you are taking a short trip to the park, or a trip across the country, always make sure you have the essentials covered. It's a good idea to not only have your dog micro-chipped but also for them to be wearing a collar with accurate contact information on the ID tag. Even the best-behaved dogs can get lost and having their collars on can ensure your dog gets returned to you should they escape.

In addition, be sure to have water and a bowl with you as well as some extra treats. Many dogs get excited when they go for a car ride, making them thirstier (and hungrier) than usual. Even though you only intended to go on a short trip, things happen, cars break down, and unfortunately, accidents happen too. Be prepared for the "what ifs."

Lastly, and perhaps most importantly, never leave a dog in the car unattended. This doesn't just go for the hot summer and cold winter months. A dog can get anxious when unaccompanied, and anything can happen, from them having an accident in the car, to destructing your seats, to even moving the gear shift! Even five minutes is too long. If you have to go into a store "really quick" be safe and drop your dog off at home first, or have someone stay with your dog to ensure they are safe.

Happy travels!

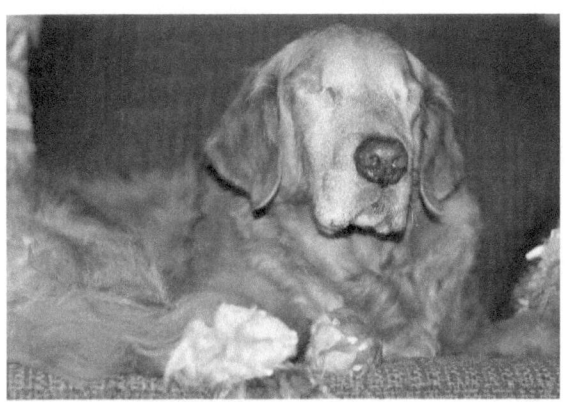

Chapter 10-Don't Move That!

While blind dogs can often find their way around, there are many things we can do to make their life even easier.

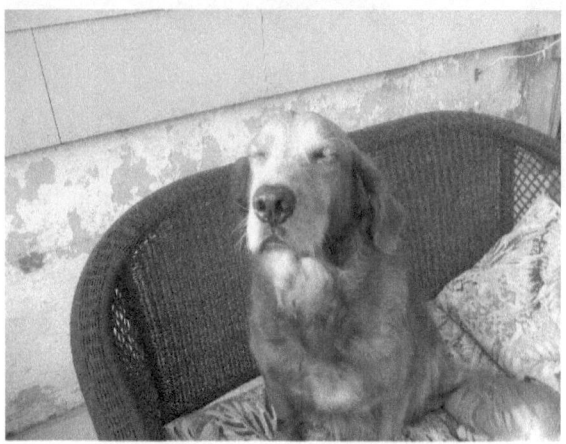

If you've ever owned a blind dog, you may have been amazed at how well they can move through the house. Sometimes it seems that they do so effortlessly.

There are certain things, however, that can throw them off and moving the furniture or, without realizing it, introducing something new to the home are just a couple of those things!

There are also little things you CAN do to ensure their safety the best that you can.

For instance, many types of furniture have pointy edges. While this might not be something you'd ordinarily mind, at a dog's height, these can be damaging!

Pieces of furniture, such as coffee tables are at about the same height as a dog, and if you've ever accidentally bumped into one, you know how badly they can hurt, especially if you are walking a little fast!

Yes, I've done this and have experienced it firsthand. Foolishly thinking I could walk flawlessly in the dark, one night, I walked right into the edge of the bed and gave myself a three-inch scar on my leg. (Yes, it hurt and yes, I screamed quite a few obscenities)! Now imagine your dog bumping into that same edge! At their height, they can easily get a large cut that same size on their cute, little, furry face!

I learned this the hard way when Goldie was racing around (as she normally does when she smells food)! Because she was not focusing on her surroundings, she bumped her head on one of these corners.

Thankfully, she did get right back up and head for the kitchen, however, I noticed she had a good size lump on her head that took a few weeks to heal!

The good news is, fixing this issue and preventing it from happening again is simple.

Home improvement stores sell little foam bumpers that have self-adhesive tape on the back. Some brands are already shaped like corners, and some you have to cut-to-fit, but both work well. Simply place these on each corner. They are life-savers for your dog (and possibly for you too)!

Also, moving the furniture can be detrimental to your dog! When your blind pet is used to where everything is, moving furniture even an inch can throw them off. While those of us who can see might not notice a huge difference, blind dogs truly have their surroundings fully mapped out!

As an example, Goldie has her favorite couch. She knows how to get on by herself and every time lays in her favorite spot.

When she wants to jump off, she goes to her second favorite spot across the room. She knows exactly how to get there without error.

Silly me, moved the furniture just a little, thinking "well, it's only a few inches." Yes, it was. However, those few inches were enough for Goldie to become confused.

She jumped on the couch but did not land in her favorite spot. She couldn't find the armrest where she normally rests her head.

Therefore, when she got off of the couch, she couldn't quite figure out where she was in the room or had to get to her other favorite spot. She was completely disoriented.

Another example, area rugs! As my dogs get older, they have a little bit of trouble walking on tile floors. So, to help matters, I purchased a few area rugs, thinking I was doing the "right thing."

It's easy to forget how small differences can make such big confusion for blind dogs!

After I made sure they were strategically placed, I put Goldie on a leash and walked her over the area rugs.

She put one foot on and stopped dead in her tracks. The confusion on her face was evident, and she refused to take another step. It took a few days before she understood the layout of the house again.

One of the new area rugs is in the kitchen, leading to the smaller, old area rug that she is used to. The smaller rug is right by the door she uses to go outside.

Since putting down the NEW area rug, she didn't understand where the door was and would slowly try to step outside, even though we weren't quite by the door yet.

Again, I had to "show" her, by gradually guiding her on the leash. As we approached the door, I took her foot and helped her "feel" the outside. Now, she finally caught on that there is another rug to walk on!

See? These little details that would ordinarily seem to be no big deal are a VERY big deal to a blind dog!

While I'm on the subject, keep your dog's blindness in mind when decorating for the holidays.

Many people put up a big tree at Christmas time. Of course, during the year this big tree is not anywhere in your house. Think about what would happen if your pet accidentally stumbled into it. At best, they might bounce back and turn around. At worst, they can knock the tree over, along with all of the ornaments and possibly injure themselves in the process.

It's wonderful to decorate, but it might be a good idea to put the tree in a place your dog won't normally go or buy a small tree to place atop of a table that IS usually in your home. Try to get into the mindset and height of your blind pet and predict possible obstacles if you can.

Lastly, if your blind dog has trouble finding the water bowl on their own, you might want to try one of the water fountains for dogs. They make a noise which might help your blind dog find it. Alternatively, you can try having an area rug leading to the water bowl. Since dogs also feel around with their feet, they may be able to find it, sniffing and walking along the area rug. Their own little red carpet to the water bowl! (Well, any color will do)!

One more tip. If your dog has been used to sleeping on the bed with you, they still can. However, one word of caution. It is very easy for them to fall off and can be very dangerous to them. You can buy a fairly inexpensive bed rail that folds down when you are not using it. Just make sure it is high enough so that your dog can't trip over it when moving around on the bed. If you find it still not safe, perhaps buy a cushy dog bed, or even one that is slightly raised and place it right by your own bed. They won't feel alone and will still be very close to you.

In fact, Goldie loves her dog bed so much now that one night I came home a little past her bedtime and found she had ventured from the living room into her bed in the bedroom and tucked herself in!

Chapter 11 - Introducing People

It can be a wonderful experience meeting new people and their pets, but to a blind dog, that meeting can be a little scary!

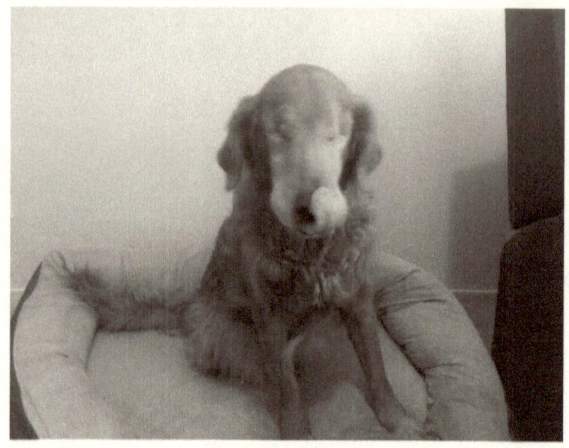

Goldie is a very complacent, lovable and friendly dog. However, every dog has their threshold and fear factor, and I'm aware of that fact.

While she typically loves everyone she meets, she has still hesitated just a bit upon meeting newcomers.

What many people do is quickly walk up to her and put both hands out for her to smell. Of course, letting them sniff your hand is a good rule of thumb, however, BOTH hands can easily startle a blind dog.

Two hands mean two different scents are coming from two different directions. A little bit of sensory overload can cause a blind dog to become perplexed.

So now, when newcomers want to meet Goldie, I ask them to let her sniff just one hand. Once she can do that, she is fine.

I have to put this in here as a little warning. It's important to let people know your dog is blind. I hate always to bring attention to that fact, but it's really to keep your dog and the person safe.

There are bandanas sold that you can attach to their leash that say "blind dog" or something similar. These are truly a great idea. I experienced a minor episode that could have ended up tragically!

One afternoon, I walked to the Goldie to the park and in the park was a bunch of people. In one corner was a Mom and five of her young children.

Before I could avoid the situation, the five kids ran over, and when they saw that Goldie had no eyes, some began screaming "She has no eyes!" and others wanted to pet her. My instincts told me to leave because five kids running up to Goldie and screaming at her was not a good thing.

I saw her body stiffen up displaying that she was getting nervous. Shielding her from the kids with my own body, one kid reached around and tried to POKE Goldie's eye sockets in!

Thankfully, I put my hands over Goldie's face and guarded the rest of her, not allowing the kids to get close. Finally, their mother called them away.

I shudder to think what COULD have happened if I couldn't shield Goldie in time. Screaming and poking is not something she is used to!

Another woman in the park approached me and said even she was nervous for me as trying to control five young kids that were NOT my own AND my dog was not easy.

Thus, having a bandana might have alerted the mother that perhaps she could have kept her children away until asking if it was okay for them to pet my dog. Though a potentially dangerous situation was avoided, the thought of what could have happened is a scary one.

It made me think, however, that it might not be only kids who are not sure about how to approach a blind dog. Prior to Goldie, I didn't have much experience with a dog who couldn't see. I had no idea what obstacles lie before them. When you don't see it first-hand, it's easy to overlook certain things—normal things—that we take for granted. I'm guilty of it as well.

If someone is racing toward us, we are aware of it because we see it coming. We can prepare ourselves for how to react. If someone puts their hands on our faces, we see it. We can see children playing and screaming and can generally ascertain what it is they are screaming about.

Now close your eyes and imagine not being able to open them. How would you feel if someone rushed at you? How would you feel if you heard loud and unfamiliar noises but didn't know where they were coming from, or what they were? It might not be as frightening now, because you have the ability to open your eyes and see for yourself. But try to imagine you couldn't. It's a frightening feeling. And I imagine that is how Goldie and other dogs like Goldie feel.

That is one of the reasons for writing this book. Of course, I wanted to tell Goldie's story. I wanted others to know that a blind dog can prosper, especially those who are indecisive about whether a blind dog has quality of life. I can say with utmost certainty, they do. I really wanted to drive that fact home after hearing people's negative and untrue opinions as I was deciding what to do regarding Goldie's surgery.

But I also wanted to bring awareness to both children and adults about certain things to be mindful of when approaching a blind dog. While blind dogs can still be confident and have independence, there are thresholds for situations they can handle. They may get spooked easily. They may not react in the best manner if a child, adult or another animal races to them. They can easily get frightened in hectic situations and where there is a lot of activity.

This isn't to say they don't like to explore. Some do. Goldie does. I recall taking her to a dog-related event here in town. Goldie absolutely loves attention and I figured she was bored of me after seeing mostly me every single day! Still, I worried about how she would react amongst a lot of people and other dogs.

She did wonderfully! She greeted everyone and her tail didn't stop wagging. She did, however, voice a few growls here and there when dogs approached her quickly. Thankfully, it was easy to put a stop to that by just telling the owners to let her approach and sniff their dogs first. That is where I learned about the bandana that says "Blind Dog" on it, and I think that is a great idea. Or at least it's a start. I believe the second part of that should be bringing awareness to all about how to react around a blind dog. And this goes for adults and children.

It only takes a few moments to talk to a child and explain to them how to approach a blind dog (or really any dog for that matter). Explaining why a dog may behave a certain way can mean the difference between a pleasant experience or a traumatic circumstance.

A few months after I met those children in the park who were racing at Goldie and trying to poke at her, I had what I thought would be a similar experience. Three young boys were climbing trees and screaming loudly. Just kids being kids. My first reaction was to turn around because I didn't want Goldie to get frightened again. As I was about to turn, the boys quieted down, climbed down from the trees and asked if they could pet Goldie. Still a little concerned, I explained to them that she is super friendly, but also blind and to allow her to approach them. They did, and it was a successful introduction. Once Goldie was able to sniff them out and, in her mind, take control of the situation, she was at ease. Her body relaxed, her tail wagged and she let them pet her. It took two seconds to explain to the boys and they were compassionate and gentle with her. That's all it takes!

The same rule applies to meeting new dogs. Of course, we can't quite explain a blind dog's situation to another dog, however, we can explain it to a dog owner. Goldie adjusts fairly well to calm dogs. But, when young dogs or dogs that are full of energy approach her, I hear the low growl coming from Goldie.

It is scary for her when anyone comes racing at her without warning. Therefore, when introducing a new dog, I only do so if they appear to be calm and controlled. I happen to adore rambunctious dogs. However, Goldie does not, and I completely understand that fact.

If I find that a dog has way too much energy, I politely tell the owner that I prefer the dogs not to meet. I'd rather not have an altercation and a potentially injured dog (or dogs)!

Chapter 12-Ginger!

Now and then, we are thrown a miracle. If we are lucky, we also get an angel.

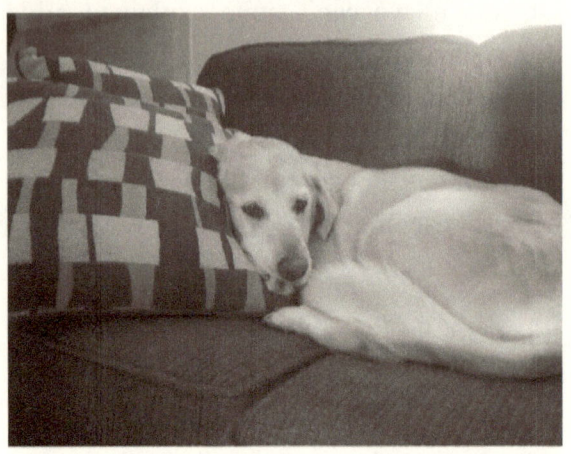

Speaking of introducing new dogs, a few months after we settled in at our new home, Goldie still appeared to be in the mourning stage over Duke.

She was happy being outside and exploring, however, inside the house, she seemed lonely. She lost interest in her toys, and while I tried to amuse her the best I could, I felt it was time for her to have a friend.

This is a personal decision for all owners of blind dogs. You have to gauge your dog's reaction when another dog approaches. Some dogs may feel the interaction is too overwhelming and their personal space and safety are being violated.

With Goldie, I already knew I would need a calm dog, but she had always been good with other dogs. I just had to find the right fit. That part was my sole mission. Making sure that I didn't just adopt any dog. This one had to be special for Goldie.

The Golden retriever rescue in town is an amazing organization, and I have adopted from them in the past.

I checked daily and contacted them, alerting them of my situation and that I'd need a special kind of dog to be Goldie's new friend. I initially wanted a male dog, since Duke was a male. My thought process was that perhaps that would be best for Goldie.

The rescue group was wonderful, keeping me posted about dogs that came in for adoption that seemed to match the description I had been seeking.

After a few weeks, they thought they had the perfect match, a young male duck tolling retriever who was super friendly.

I was very excited because I used to have a Duck Toller, named Toffee and I love their charismatic personalities.

As with every dog I have adopted, I could not wait to meet him. Early one morning, I took Goldie to meet him, and they seemed to get along!

The problem happened when we got home. This sweetheart of a dog was full of energy! He was able to jump on top of the counters and tables with all four paws in one hop.

And he wasn't shy about jumping very close to Goldie.

He barked often and was very lovable to Goldie, but very loud for her. Once again, I heard Goldie's low growl and saw Goldie trying to run away from him, bumping into things as she did. That was the only indication I needed that she was not comfortable with her new friend.

Sadly, it was not a good match. I loved him. However, I had to make sure both dogs would get along well and didn't want either to be miserable or worse, harmed! Even if they never fought, if I wasn't there when Goldie would try to run from him, she could have easily gotten hurt.

Back to the drawing board.

About a week later, the rescue called and said they had an older dog; however, it was a female. I thought a male would get along better with Goldie but decided to give it a try.

Off we went in the car, and this time, the two dogs met at Bass Pro. Their introduction was very similar to how Goldie and Duke had behaved upon their first meeting.

Ginger was a white golden retriever, who was about nine or ten years old when we met her.

She had the typical bumps that accompany senior dogs, but overall, had a clean bill of health!

Gentle as can be, she slowly walked up to Goldie They shook hands in their canine matter and then sat next to each other as if they were getting together for lunch.

I knew this was the one! Ginger and Goldie were the PERFECT match!

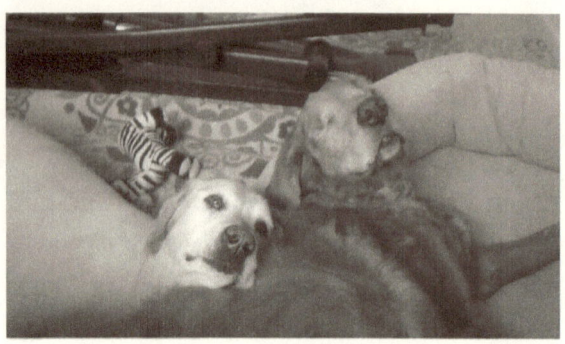

The ride home was a cinch. I was a little apprehensive about it as I was by myself. Having two dogs, who had just met, in the car while I was driving could be scary, especially if they began to have a tiff. Fortunately, they both laid down and didn't make a peep!

When we arrived home, Ginger was a little more hyper than she led on, running through the house, jumping OVER the couches and exploring her new home with pure excitement! Goldie didn't seem to mind, as Ginger was still calm around her, almost as if Ginger sensed Goldie preferred it that way.

There was not even much of a training curve with Ginger. She had a few accidents in the house, and I could tell in her previous home she was a counter surfer as she almost grabbed a pizza off of the counter! She also lived by the rule, "if it's in the house, it's mine!" I could see by the condition of her teeth that this dog must have chewed everything and anything!

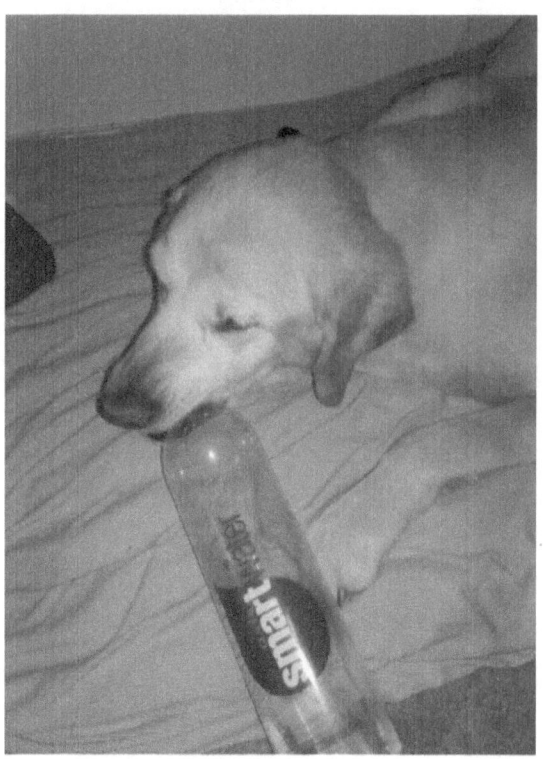

However, within what seemed like just days, she acclimated and started going to the bathroom outside and learned what she could and couldn't chew. Hence, there are toy chests all over the house filled with safe toys which has kept Ginger occupied…and my furniture quite safe!

I also noticed one very important thing. Goldie was slowly losing her depression. She began playing with toys again, wagging her tail more and becoming more energetic. She was truly enjoying Ginger's company.

The two are now inseparable. They sleep together during the day and at night, nestled right next to each other.

Ginger helps Goldie around the house and alerts me when she hears Goldie shuffling around.

While sometimes Ginger might lead her a little bit in the wrong direction, she does sort of guide Goldie with her own body so that Goldie can follow her.

I couldn't be happier with the two. Watching them together is some of the most peaceful moments of my day.

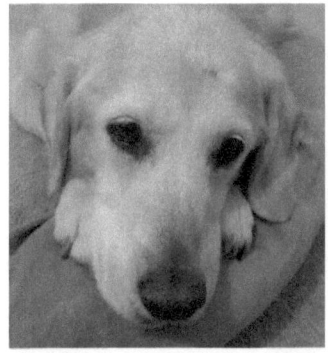

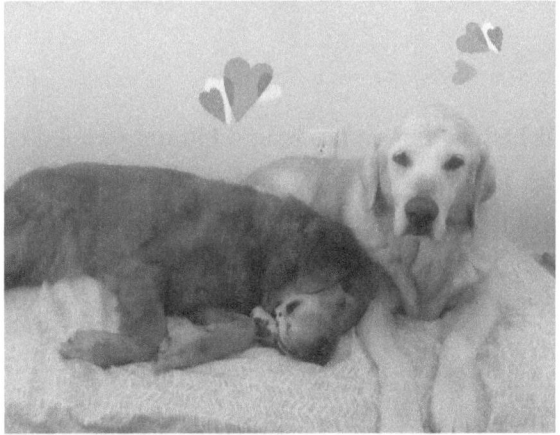

Chapter 13-Blind dogs CAN swim!

Challenges come when we least expect it. It's important to try to stay calm, stay focused and think outside the box. Sometimes, what we think is impossible is indeed very possible!

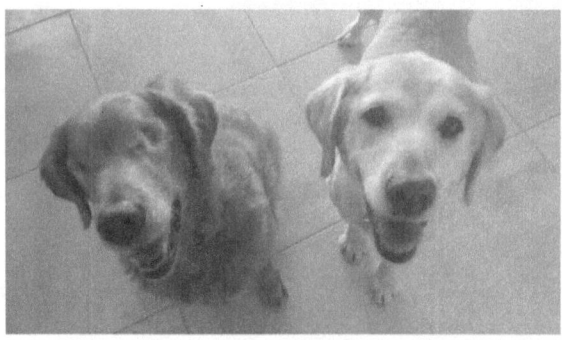

When it rains, it pours and Goldie seemed to be needing an umbrella! Everything was going beautifully with Goldie and Ginger. Finally, life was back on track and everyone was adjusting to their new lives, including myself!

The old cliché holds true. Actually, a few clichés hold true. Always appreciate the little things and never take anything for granted.

Goldie had made such progress dealing with her blindness, losing her brother Duke, moving across the country and living life in an entirely new house in an entirely new state.

As luck would have it, she proved her genes were real in being a golden retriever and woke up one day in a lot of pain.

I panicked as I dialed the emergency center which cleared the way for me to rush Goldie in. Goldie could not walk and groaned whenever I moved her.

Once I arrived, the veterinary technicians rushed out and wheeled Goldie into the vet's office in a gurney. Watching my little trooper lay motionless was upsetting beyond belief.

Where was my little barker who loved to play? I think I grew a bunch of gray hairs as I sat in the waiting room of the emergency center while they took X-rays.

Thinking the worst, but hoping for the best, I tried to remember each day over the previous week, and only one instance stood out, which was Goldie tripping on the driveway and falling. It didn't seem like a major ordeal at the time, because while Goldie maneuvered around fairly well, she still had her moments when she'd bump into things or trip. It never bothered her before.

Since I was at an emergency center, the wait was longer than usual, and I sat for three hours trying only to think the best and keeping my imagination from growing wild.

Admittedly, I felt I was going to lose my mind as all I wanted to do is get my dog back and hug her until she felt better.

Finally, after three hours, the doctor came in and told me Goldie had very bad hip dysplasia. Not the news I wanted to hear, but better than what could have been.

Golden retrievers are prone to cancer, and that was the first thing that entered my mind. So, hearing that Goldie just needed pain medications was still music to my ears. My Goldie would be going home with me that day after all.

I didn't know how quickly the pain meds would take effect, however, the next day, she was able to stand on her own and even walk, albeit slowly, however much better than the previous day!

It is these small bittersweet miracles for which I am thankful. Of course, I don't want any of my dogs actually to have hip dysplasia, but there are things to help manage pain. Some simpler than others.

To start, I immediately decided to get artificial grass in the yard. Here in Vegas, the yard was complete rock. Not easy, nor comfortable to walk on. Goldie had a tough time walking on it and would often trip, or sometimes her hind legs would give out.

Since Goldie needed a level ground, I reasoned that artificial grass would be the best option. Luckily, it was.

No longer did Goldie stumble walking on it and she was once again able to roll around and play on the level and soft ground.

The second thing I did was search the Internet for swimming facilities for dogs. I didn't even know if such a thing existed! I was thrilled when I found one in town that wasn't too far away.

After speaking with the Kathy, the owner of Canine Bodywork and Aquatics, I explained Goldie's blindness and asked if it would be a problem.

To my knowledge, Goldie had never swum before. I had no idea how she would react. Contrary to popular belief, not ALL goldens enjoy swimming! I've had several, and only one ever mastered the pool and one that tolerated it. The rest were terrified of water.

Now, imagine a blind dog being submerged in water if they had never swum before.

I was a little worried she wouldn't react well, but if it would help her hips, I had to give it a try.

The owner explained that Goldie could wear a life preserver and that she would be in the pool with Goldie the entire time.

So, at the first available appointment, Goldie and I ventured out.

The facility was clean, and the padding on the floor was much like that of a yoga mat. It was spongy, making it easier for dogs to walk on.

We ventured up the padded ramp and was greeted by Kathy, along with soothing meditation music and the relaxing aroma of essential oils.

I had a really good feeling about this.

Kathy greeted Goldie and Goldie wagged her tail nonstop, loving the new attention.

We spoke for a while, and after we all got acquainted, we put on Goldie's life preserver.

There was a little step to get into the pool, and we helped Goldie find it by using the good old commands that work wonderfully, "step up!"

We slowly lowered Goldie into the pool and Kathy held onto Goldie the entire time.

We watched Goldie closely. She was a little stressed and breathing a bit heavier than normal, but nothing that showed she was panicking. She was getting used to things.

It was apparent that Goldie had never swum before, as she didn't understand the free buoyancy underneath her legs. Like a baby's first time in a pool, Goldie began kicking her front and back legs around, splashing water all over the walls and floor.

Within a few minutes, her breathing was more relaxed. However, she still did not master swimming. She was soaked, I was soaked, and the floor was soaked!

However, she seemed to be enjoying the gravitational freedom. There was no impact on her legs, so the water was the perfect thing for her.

Once her session was over, Kathy helped her out of the pool and ended the therapy with a wonderful massage for Goldie.

By the time we left, Goldie was rolling over on her back, paws grasping at her masseuse in her typical fashion, as if to say "more, more!"

By the second or third session, Goldie's swimming ability had greatly improved.

She looked forward to going and knew where we were going each time. When we pulled into the parking lot, she began to get anxious in the car and couldn't wait to go swimming with her new instructor!

Funny enough, she knew which door to go in without me needing to guide her. This, after just one session!

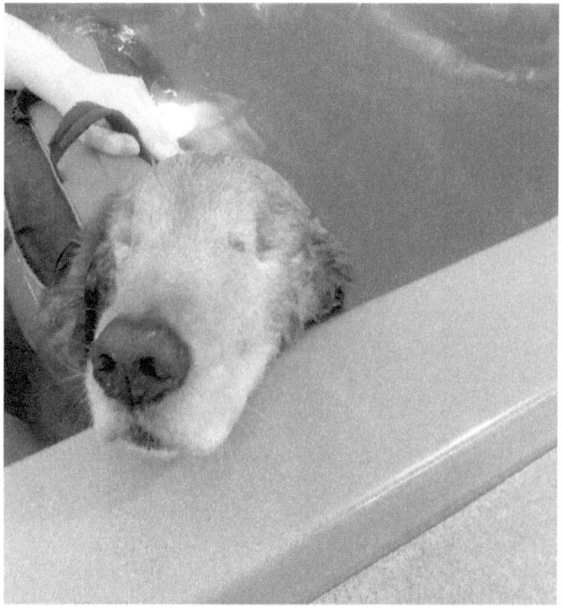

She was Kathy's first blind client, and it was Goldie's first blind swim or, from what I could tell, the only time she had ever swum!

This little dog with so many issues continued to amaze me. She had overcome so many obstacles in life and continued to persevere and press on.

When I first got the news that Goldie's eyes needed to be enucleated, I didn't even know if she'd be able to go on daily walks again, no less swim.

Yet there she was, swimming, and swimming well! No more messy splashing!

But, I say to her anyway- make a splash Goldie. You've earned it!

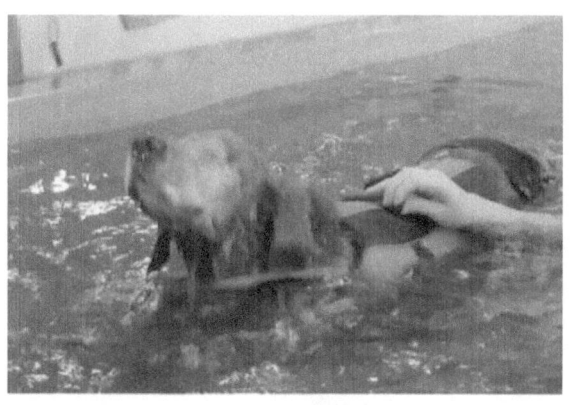

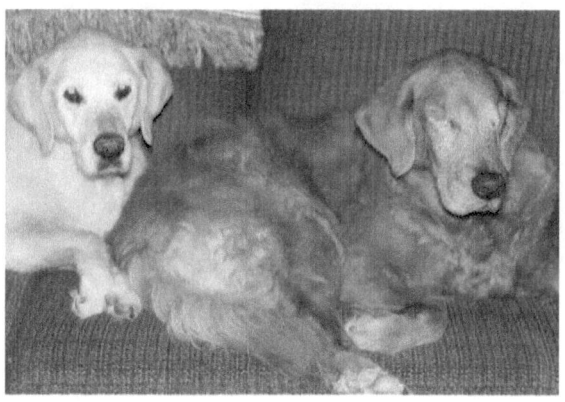

Chapter 14-A Thread of Awareness

Just like with many fully abled dogs, sometimes they become sick. One illness, however, that is difficult to determine in blind dogs is Vestibular disease. I wanted to add this in here because while Vestibular can strike any dog, the main symptom is not as obvious in a dog without eyes!

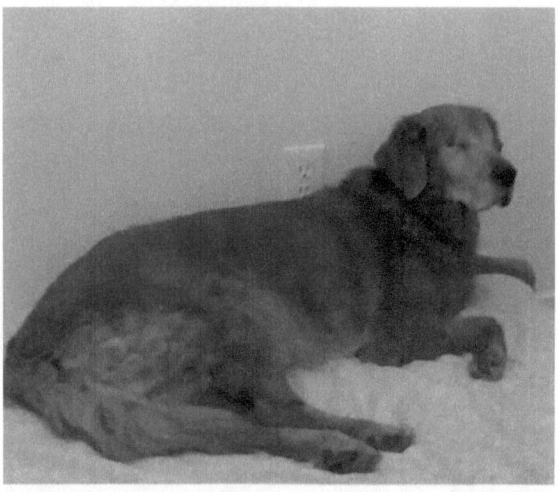

As our dogs begin the aging process, we notice gradual changes in their activity levels or even slight differences in their personality.

They may move a little slower, or not want to go on long walks like they usually do.

What we don't count on is our dogs having a wonderful day, only to see a major difference only a few hours later.

While many illnesses can come on suddenly, one that is frightening to see is this illness.

It is a disease that often affects older dogs and can occur instantaneously.

At first, it is difficult to determine just what is going on with your pet. They may walk super slow, or worse, not be able to walk at all. They may drag their legs, or walk in circles. You may notice they tilt their head to one side and their face might even be droopy. There are varying levels of intensity with this disease, as some dogs suffer from nausea, and won't eat or drink. They may appear like they want to but seem to be confused as to how to do so!

In addition, you will most likely notice a very distinct trait of this disease—their eyes will move back and forth quickly. For dogs without eyes, you need to take a closer look.

You obviously will not see their eyes moving. However, their eye muscles will still move back and forth in a very noticeable manner!

Some of these symptoms mimic that of a stroke, so if this happens to your dog, it is best to get them examined by your veterinarian immediately for proper care in either case.

If determined that it is Vestibular, there is a light at the end of the tunnel, even though seeing your dog in this distressed state is indeed very frightening.

Fortunately, in most instances, this disease goes away on its own, usually within one day, up to two weeks.

It can be caused by an inner ear infection, idiopathic reasons, and in some cases, there could be a more serious issue.

Vestibular is similar to vertigo, in that your dog cannot make spatial judgments, and they are very dizzy. If they are nauseous, they will not want to eat or drink. In that case, your veterinarian can administer anti-nausea medicine. Also, if your pooch is dehydrated, your vet can administer fluid under your dog's skin to keep them hydrated.

While there is no cure, if your vet finds that an inner ear infection is evident, they may administer medicine to cure it.

The best thing to do during your pup's recovery time is to keep them in a confined, quiet area where they can't fall or get hurt. Keep them away from stairs and pools. You may find you need to bring them food and water if they can't make it to their feeding area on their own. When you need to take them outside, there are harnesses that make it easier for you to lift them, especially if you have a larger dog.

Take notice to make sure that your pet is improving. If you find that they seem to be getting worse, let your veterinarian know. Otherwise, try to stay calm and patient. Hopefully, within in a few days, you'll see marked improvement!

This happened to Goldie, and I thought for sure that the end was near or that her hip dysplasia had gotten the better of her. She couldn't stand up, her back legs dragged behind her.

Her head tilted to one side, and while she wasn't wincing in pain, it was painfully obvious that she was certainly not having a good day.

After a very sleepless night, I rushed her to the veterinarian first thing, and that is where he pointed out the rapid movement in her eye muscles.

Since a dog I had owned previously had suffered from vestibular, I knew the outcome was a positive one and breathed a very, very big sigh of relief!

Yes, it is difficult to witness a dog suffering from this disease, however, knowing that more often than not, it is temporary takes the anxiety away. At least a little. I can't help but be a worrier by nature, so I wasn't completely happy until Goldie was back to her barking, funny self!

When I say that Goldie is my hero those are not just words.

What I didn't mention in previous chapters was that during all of this I had been diagnosed with DCIS on my 44th birthday. Not quite a happy birthday! So, in essence, I was coping (or at least trying to cope) with my divorce, Goldie's blindness and surgery, my surgery and sadly Duke's passing.

Keep in mind the situations weren't so sad that it would almost be ironically funny as they all happened on holidays or special occasions — Goldie's eye enucleation on St Patrick's Day, my diagnosis on my birthday and Duke's passing on Valentine's Day.

Also, I moved across the country and changed jobs, a positive but challenging major life change. It was a lot for me to handle but I looked at my little sidekick Goldie and realized that aside from the DCIS, divorce and job change, she had been going to the same things I had.

After all, she was the one who lost her sight, and she also lost her brother Duke.

She moved across the country with me, exploring unknown cities and states that she had obviously never seen before. She moved into a house that she had never seen before either and had the courage to accept it all and put her trust and faith in me.

By watching her, it in turn, made me strong and then I realized that if this sweet dog was able to persevere, then I had to learn by her example and do the same.

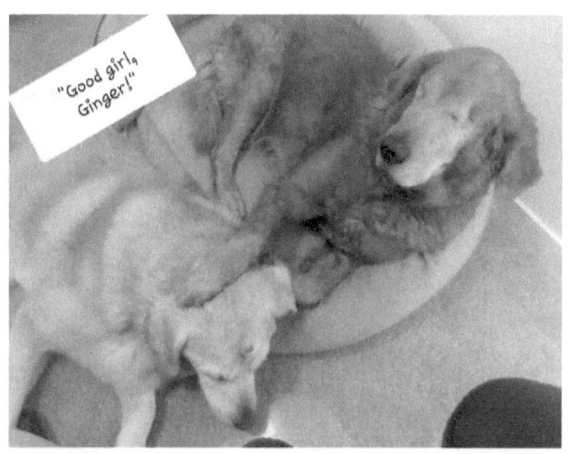

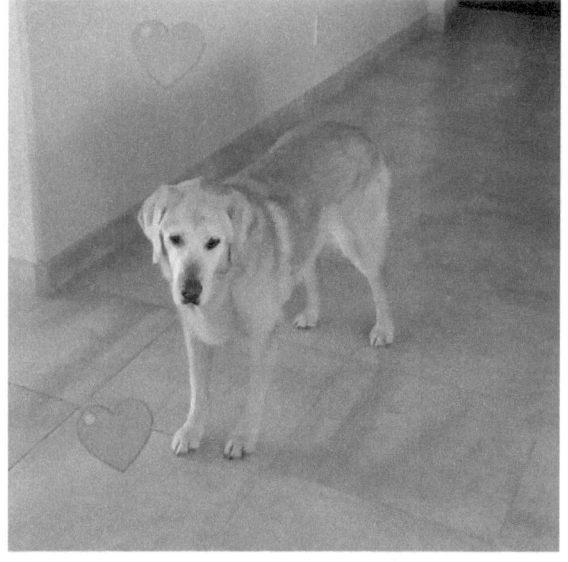

Extras to remember

Just remember, blind dogs can do a lot of things fully-abled dogs can do.

They can enjoy a nice swing in the fresh air.

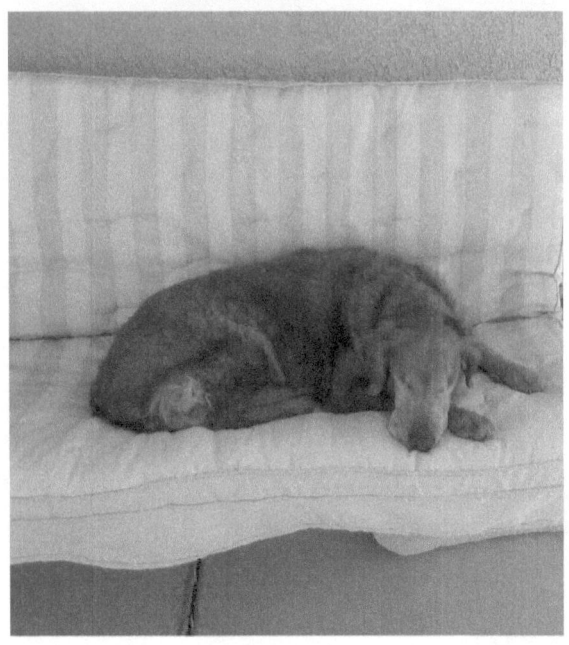

They still have expressions.

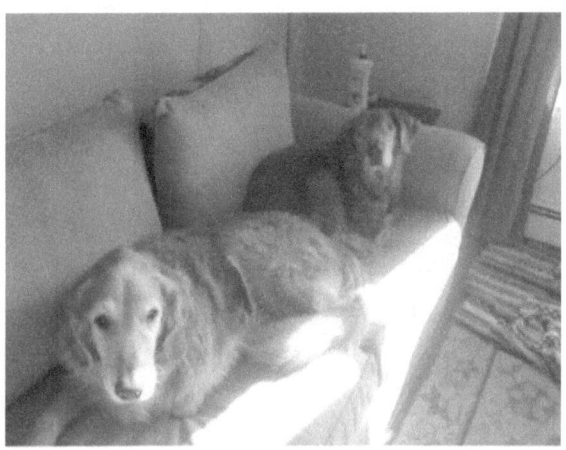

They still roll around in the grass!

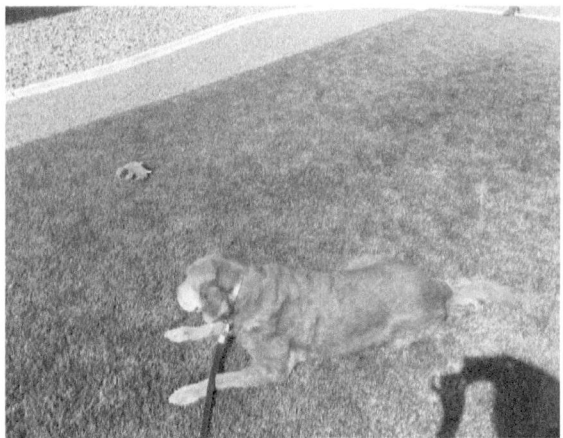

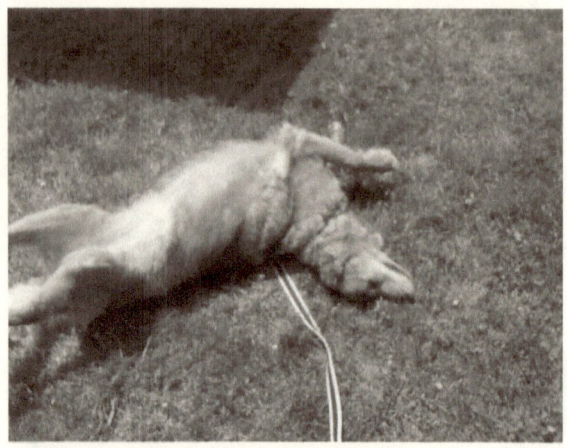

They still celebrate holidays!

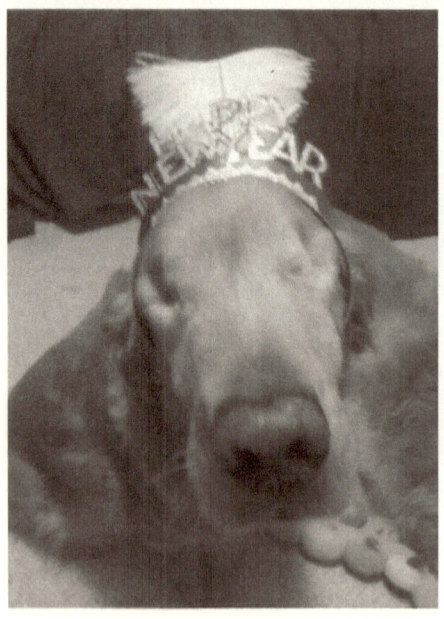

And they still LOVE to snuggle!

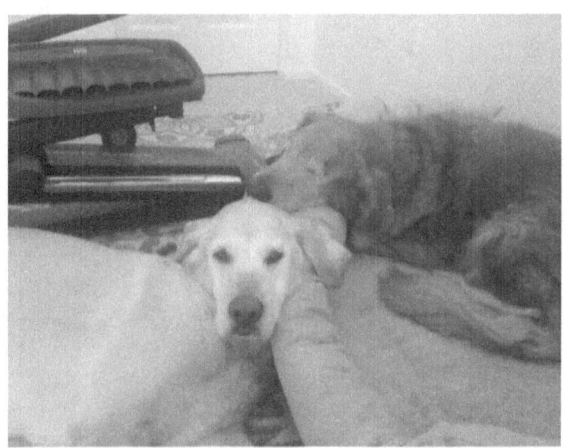

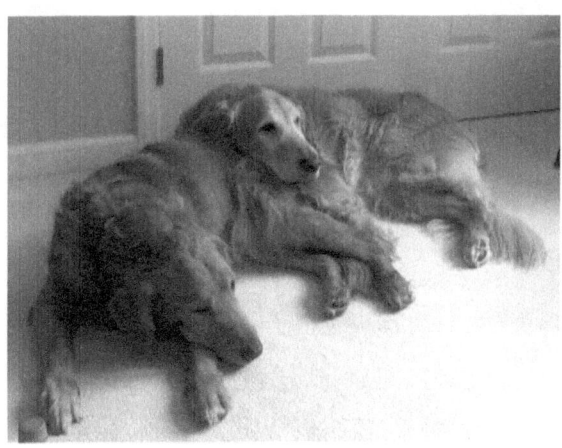

Remember, they are still the same lovable dog they were when they had vision. They see you, just in their own special way. With their heart.

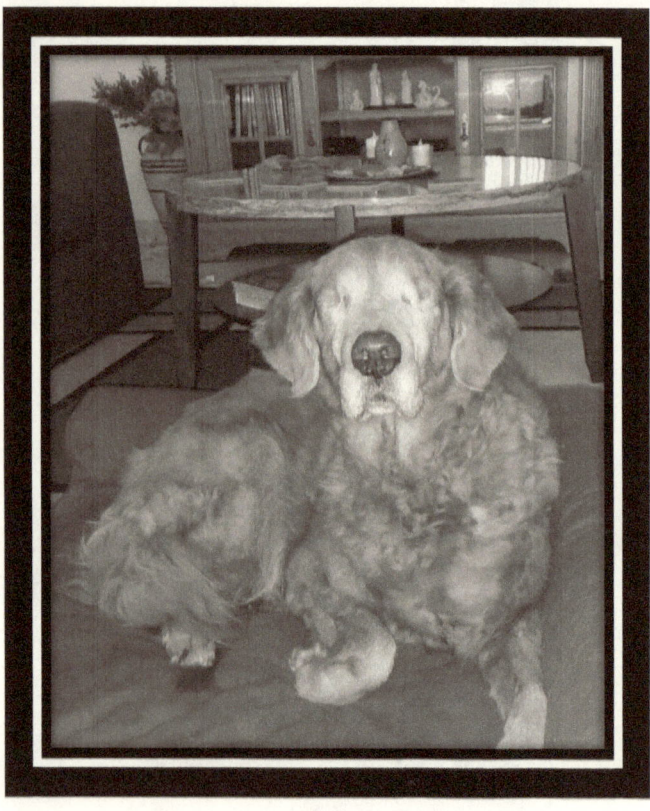

If asked if I would ever adopt a blind dog, my answer is a resounding YES! Goldie successfully moved across the country, played tourist in each state, learned how to swim, made new friends and thrived. I've stated this fact numerous times and I'll say it again. Goldie is my hero. She is the one that shows that anything is possible. She changed my mind to possibly help disabled dogs in the future, something I never thought I could do.

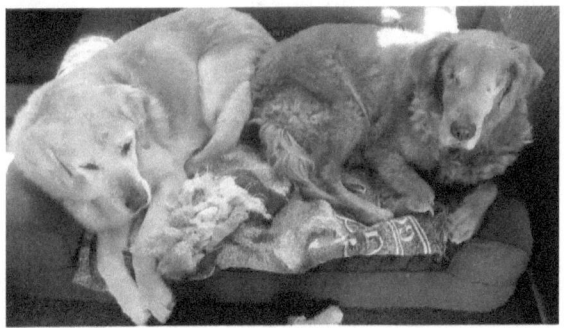

Dog Sitters

This is just a little extra. I don't travel too often, but when I do, I tend to write a novel just on care instructions alone!

If you worry as much as I do, perhaps you write a novel of your own on how to care for your pet in your absence!

Throughout the years, I've refined my instructions and have strived to cover all of the "what ifs."

Since sometimes it's necessary to get away, I thought this checklist might help fellow dog lovers!

What Every Dog Sitter Needs to Know

Don't tell your pooch, but sometimes you might want to take a vacation without them. Yikes!

It can be stressful, but there are things you can do to make it a little easier. If you have a reputable pet sitter that can come to the house, you'll want your pet sitter to be as prepared as possible to make them feel more confident while watching your pets. It will also make you feel relieved having all bases covered.

Here is some information your dog sitter will want to know about your fur-baby:

Feeding Schedule and how much, including daily snacks.

Any allergies or medications

Dog(s) fears or quirks

- For blind dogs, explain to the sitter the commands or the tricks you use to help your pup out of a tight spot. Let them know if your dog needs a leash to go outside (as Goldie does) or are they capable of going potty without one.
- For Goldie, she needs to be shown her water bowl. If this is the case with your blind dog, let the sitter know this so that your dog doesn't go thirsty in your absence!

Potty breaks (times and intervals between each).

Should your dog be exercised?

Vet and vet emergency phone numbers, locations and hours.

Phone number of where to reach you.

Bedtime – is your dog the type who knows their bedtime and starts to get antsy summoning you to bed as the clock strikes that hour? If so, your sitter will want to know this!

Along those same lines, where does the dog(s) sleep?

If you cannot find a sitter, you might have to board your dog in a kennel.

Hopefully, your pooch won't mind spending a few days away from family to discover new and exciting territories!

When choosing the kennel for your dog, there are some additional factors to consider:

Cost: Make sure that the final amount due meets your budget.

Scheduling time: Find out how much time in advance you need to schedule your pet' stay.

Dog interaction: Does this facility have a play area for all of the dogs to get to know each other? This can be a great advantage if you have a dog who loves social activities, but some dogs don't play well with others. You can let the facility know your preference.

Is someone always on premises? If there's an emergency, will someone be there to bring your dog to safety?

Emergency Vet: Unfortunately, accidents happen, and sometimes healthy dogs become ill. Is there an emergency veterinarian on call and will they take appropriate action to get your dog immediate care?

What if You Can't Pick Them Up due to Your Own Emergency? Be sure to have a contingency plan in your absence in case you are delayed.

Don't forget to inquire about these details as well!

- Drop off time, Pick up time

- Is there a group Discount for more than one dog or referral discount?

- Size of Pen

- Is there access to the outdoors from your dog's pen?

- Exercise

- Cleanliness/ Temperature Controlled

- Live Cam Available?

- Will Someone administer medicines?

A few last items to bring:

- Vaccination papers

- Blanket/Toys/Beds

- Your dog's food

- Treats

- Medicines (if applicable)

On the day of drop off, try to make it a positive experience. Our dogs sense our moods and will pick up on anxiety or sadness. Try to be relaxed and upbeat. The better experience they have the first time, the less they will be frightened the next time!

~~

If you find yourself living with a blind dog and find obstacles, there are many forums online. Don't hesitate to ask your veterinarian for sound advice.

In addition, your dog will tell you more than you realize. Pay attention to their body language. What works for one blind dog might not work for another. All personalities and likes/dislikes are different. Your dog will tell you. Their way of telling you might be subtle, but watch them closely and hopefully you will be able to determine what it is that they need!

Other Books by Elizabeth Parker

Unwanted Dreams

Phobia

Evil's Door

Faces of Deception

Occupational Hazard-Perfect Lies

Final Journey: Buddys' Book

My Dog Does That!

Paw Prints in the Sand

Paw Prints in the Sand: Mission Accomplished

Hearts of Gold

Bark Out Loud!

Fur-Baby's Keepsake Book

Dog Book: It's All About the Dogs

Dogs Behaving Badly

Goldie: A Day in the Life of a Blind Dog

"Purr" Baby's Mementos Book

Passionate

Reflections on Life, Love, and Dogs

Silly Pups Coloring Book

Love of Dogs Journal – with Quotes!

The Light at the End of the Tunnel

Pet's Medical Journal

Cypress Cove

Enchanted

Peace, Love, Paws

Virtuous Victory

Blaze of Fury

Silent Redemption

Dog Baby Book: A Baby Book for your Dog

Cat Baby Book: A Baby Book for your Cat

Children's Books:

Tails From the Rainbow Bridge

Where is Cooper?

Cooper Goes to the Amusement Park

Cooper Visits a Farm

Cooper Goes White Water Rafting

Cooper Celebrates Howl-o-ween

Cooper's Festive Thanksgiving

Cooper's First Baseball Game

Cooper and the Rockin' Reindeer

Cooper Goes to a St. Patrick's Day Parade

Cooper's Big Day: A Bully, a Birthday, and a Big Surprise

Cooper Saves Easter

Cooper's Big Book of Adventures

www.ingramcontent.com/pod-product-compliance
Lightning Source LLC
Chambersburg PA
CBHW021412210526
45463CB00001B/332